Antibiotic Therapy in Urology

ANTIBIOTIC THERAPY IN UROLOGY

EDITOR
S. GRANT MULHOLLAND, M.D.
NATHAN LEWIS HATFIELD PROFESSOR AND CHAIRMAN
DEPARTMENT OF UROLOGY
JEFFERSON MEDICAL COLLEGE
OF THOMAS JEFFERSON UNIVERSITY
PHILADELPHIA, PENNSYLVANIA

Lippincott - Raven
PUBLISHERS
Philadelphia • New York

Lippincott-Raven Publishers, 227 East Washington Square, Philadelphia, Pennsylvania 19106

Made in the United States of America

Library of Congress Cataloging-in-Publication Data

Antibiotic therapy in urology / editor, S. Grant Mulholland.
p. cm.
Includes bibliographical references and index.
ISBN 0-397-51586-3
1. Urinary tract infections—chemotherapy. 2. Antibiotics.
I. Mulholland, S. Grant.
[DNLM: 1. Urogenital Diseases—drug therapy. 2. Antibiotics—therapeutic use. WJ 140 A629 1996]
RC901.8.A58 1995
616.6'0651—dc20
DNLM/DLC
for Library of Congress 95-39528

The material contained in this volume was submitted as previously unpublished material, except in the instances in which credit has been given to the source from which some of the illustrative material was derived.

Great care has been taken to maintain the accuracy of the information contained in the volume. However, neither Lippincott-Raven Publishers nor the editor can be held responsible for errors or for any consequences arising from the use of the information contained herein.

9 8 7 6 5 4 3 2 1

Contents

Contributors

Rodney U. Anderson, M.D. *Professor of Urology, Department of Urology, Stanford University School of Medicine, 300 Pasteur Drive, Stanford, California 94305; and Santa Clara Valley Medical Center, 751 South Bascom Avenue, San Jose, California 95128*

Hanna Bialkowska-Hobrzanska, M.S.G., Ph.D. *Associate Professor, Department of Microbiology and Immunology, Lawson Research Institute, The University of Western Ontario, 268 Grosvenor Street, London, Ontario N6A 4U2 Canada*

Heather J. L. Brooks, Ph.D. *Lecturer, Department of Microbiology, University of Otago, P.O. Box 56, Dunedin, New Zealand*

Culley C. Carson III, M.D. *Professor and Chairman, Division of Urology, University of North Carolina at Chapel Hill School of Medicine, 427 Burnett Womack Building, Chapel Hill, North Carolina 27599-7235*

Stacy J. Childs, M.D. *Associate Clinical Professor of Urology, Department of Urology, University of Colorado Health Sciences Center, 4200 East 9th Avenue, Denver, Colorado 80262; and Cheyenne Urological, P.C., 800 East 20th Street, Cheyenne, Wyoming 82001*

Michael Corrado, M.D. *Professor of Medicine, Seton Hall University School of Medicine, South Orange, New Jersey, 07079; President, Advanced Biologics, 80 Lambert Lane, Lambertville, New Jersey, 08530*

Joseph Del Pizzo, M.D. *Resident, Department of Urology, University of Maryland School of Medicine, 22 South Greene Street, Baltimore, Maryland 21201*

Jackson E. Fowler, Jr., M.D. *Professor of Surgery, and Chief, Division of Urology, University of Mississippi Medical Center, 1200 North State Street, Jackson, Mississippi 39216*

John V. Kryger, M.D. *Resident, Division of Urology, University of Wisconsin Hospitals and Clinics, 600 Highland Avenue, Madison, Wisconsin 53705-3236*

Robert M. Moldwin, M.D. *Assistant Professor of Urology, Albert Einstein College of Medicine; and Department of Urology, Long Island Jewish Medical Center, 270-05 76th Avenue, New Hyde Park, New York 11042*

S. Grant Mulholland, M.D. *Nathan Lewis Hatfield Professor and Chairman, Department of Urology, Jefferson Medical College of Thomas Jefferson University, College Building, Philadelphia, Pennsylvania 19107*

J. Curtis Nickel, M.D., F.R.C.S.C. *Professor, Department of Urology, Queens University, Kingston General Hospital, 64 Stuart Street, Kingston, Ontario K7L 2V7 Canada*

Lindsay E. Nicolle, M.D., F.R.C.P.C. *Professor, Departments of Medicine and Medical Microbiology, University of Manitoba, MS-675 Health Sciences Centre, 820 Sherbrook Street, Winnipeg, Manitoba R3A 1R9 Canada*

C. Lowell Parsons, M.D. *Professor of Surgery and Urology, Division of Urology, University of California in San Diego, School of Medicine, Medical Center, 200 West Arbor Drive, San Diego, California 92103-8897*

Gregor Reid, Ph.D. *Associate Professor, Departments of Surgery and Microbiology and Immunology, The University of Western Ontario, Lawson Research Institute, London, Ontario N6A 4U2 Canada*

James A. Roberts, M.D. *Professor of Urology, Department of Urology, Tulane University School of Medicine, 1430 Tulane Avenue, New Orleans, Louisiana 70112; and Tulane Regional Primate Research Center, 18703 Three Rivers Road, Covington, Louisiana 70433*

Yefim R. Sheynkin, M.D. *Chief Resident, Division of Urology, Maimonides Medical Center, 4802 10th Avenue, Brooklyn, New York 11219; and Coney Island Hospital, 2601 Ocean Parkway, Brooklyn, New York 11235*

David T. Uehling, M.D. *Professor and Chairman, Division of Urology, University of Wisconsin Hospitals and Clinics, 600 Highland Avenue, G5/339 CSC, Madison, Wisconsin 53705-3236*

Miguel Valvano, M.D. *Associate Professor, Department of Microbiology and Immunology, The University of Western Ontario, Dental Sciences Building, London, Ontario N6A 5C1 Canada*

Gilbert J. Wise, M.D. *Professor of Urology, SUNY Health Science Center of Brooklyn, 450 Clarkson Avenue, Brooklyn, New York 11203; and Director, Division of Urology, Maimonides Medical Center, 4802 10th Avenue, Brooklyn, New York 11219*

Preface

Since my residency days, I have been involved in the investigation and treatment of urinary tract infection. Years ago our understanding of urinary tract infection was poor. Basic knowledge of the pathogenesis and epidemiology of urinary tract infection was just becoming apparent in the 1960s. Our understanding of all types of urinary tract infections has increased vastly through more intense investigation. From these investigations, proper evaluation and treatment have changed markedly.

This book is devoted to the utilization of antimicrobials in the treatment of urinary tract infection. It concentrates on contemporary thought and specific areas of interest. Our intention is to include topics of special controversy that will stimulate the reader. The authors have been chosen because of their particular interest and expertise in their respective topics.

In the final chapter we discuss what might develop in the future, since rapidly advancing knowledge will change treatment methods radically over the next decade.

S. Grant Mulholland, M.D.

Acknowledgment

I would like to thank the authors for helping me put together this book on the utilization of antimicrobials in the treatment of urinary tract infections. These colleagues are old friends who have contributed over the years to the enhancement of our understanding of urinary tract infections, including its etiology, pathogenesis, evaluation, and treatment. Because of their contributions, changes and improvements in treatment have occurred, which in turn have benefited many patients.

S.G.M.

Antibiotic Therapy in Urology

Antibiotic Therapy in Urology,
edited by S. Grant Mulholland, M.D.,
Lippincott-Raven Publishers, Philadelphia © 1996.

Chapter 1

Principles of Antimicrobial Therapy

Stacy J. Childs

Department of Urology, University of Colorado Health Sciences Center, Denver, Colorado 80210; and Cheyenne Urological, P.C., Cheyenne, Wyoming, 82001

It is not known how the changing health care environment in the United States will affect the development of the specialty of urology. However, one thing is certain: urologists will always be called on to diagnose and treat complicated or life-threatening urinary tract infections (UTIs) and possibly even uncomplicated infections among high-risk patients when treatment fails or is suspected of failing in the primary care setting. Billions of dollars will be spent by the health care system in future years to evaluate and treat patients with genitourinary infections, and physicians, in all likelihood, will be asked to share the risk of caring for these patients with third-party payers or the government. It behooves us, the specialists who are considered the experts in managing urinary tract infections, to know how to diagnose and cure UTIs as expeditiously and efficiently as possible—for the benefit of the health care system as well as our own livelihood.

If the current trend continues, urologists will not be able to prolong evaluation times, gamble on a diagnosis, treat with the broadest and most expensive antimicrobial agents, and not be held accountable for outcomes. Like any field undergoing change, the specialty of urology is filled with challenges, and perhaps a re-evaluation of our education is required. Possibly medical economics and cost-to-benefit paradigms should be created and taught to residents and physicians in post-graduate programs in urology. If we urologists are to hold onto this area of expertise, we may all have to review the principles of antimicrobial therapy and create standard algorithms and protocols for patient care in the infectious arena. A suggested treatment algorithm for primary care treatment of UTIs is presented in Fig. 1.

Understanding the principles of antimicrobial therapy goes far beyond identifying infecting organisms, classifying cases as uncomplicated or complicated, and betting on the sensitivity of a particular pathogen. The

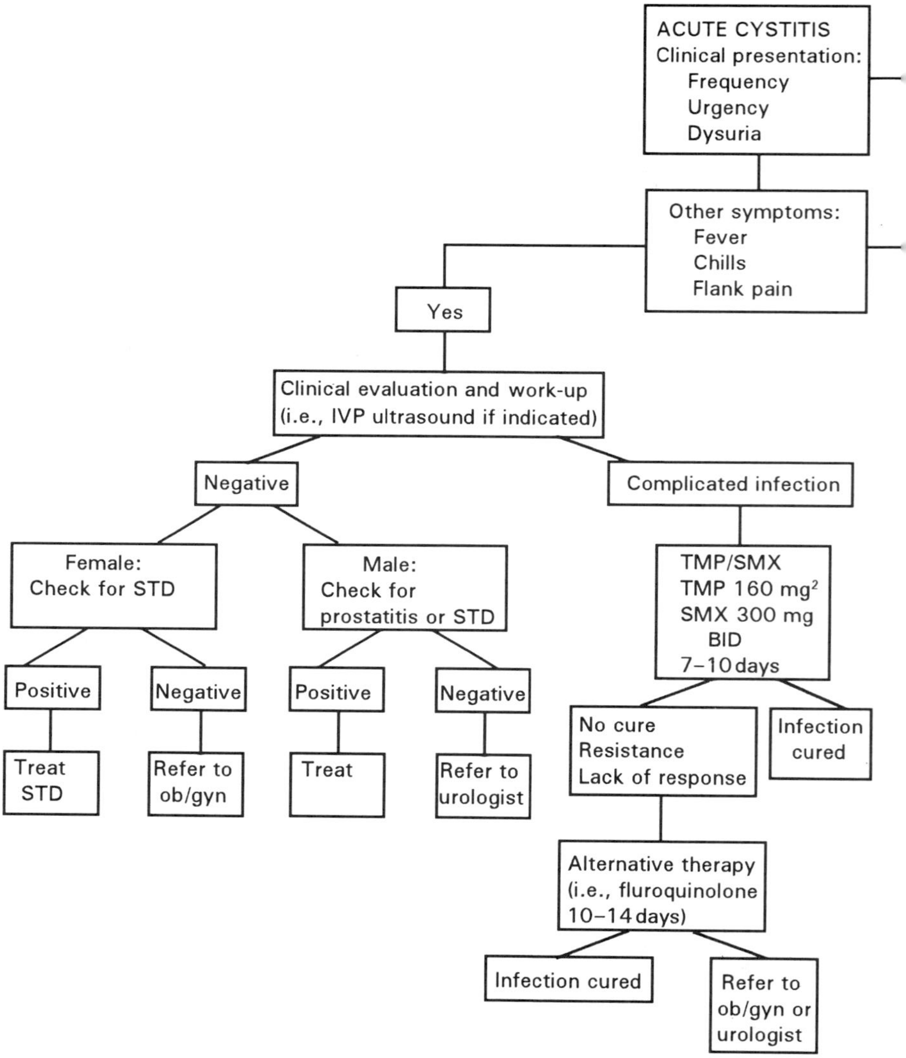

FIG. 1. Treatment algorithm for urinary tract infections

following introduction should at least stimulate some thinking relevant to the "new health care environment" and, it is hoped, motivate the members of our specialty to develop quickly an official policy to be followed by both primary care and specialty care physicians (urologists, gynecologists, pediatricians).

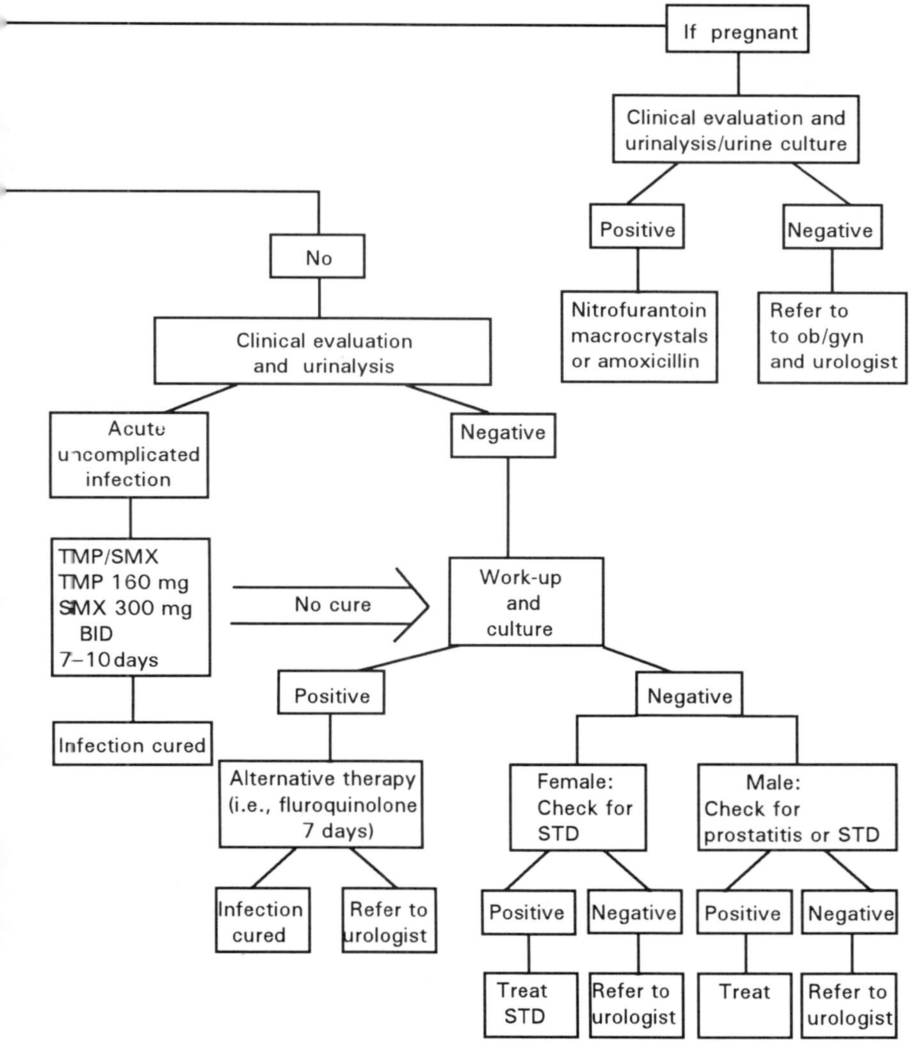

THE PATIENT AND THE PHYSICIAN AFFECT OUTCOMES

Outcomes Related to the Patient

Few physicians realize that the most important factor in the treatment of a urinary tract infection is patient compliance. If a patient does not take his or her medication, the odds are that the result is not going to be a cure. Many physicians do not understand the many aspects of compliance that influence patient behavior. One, of course, is the availability of samples in the physician's office. If sufficient samples are distributed to the patient for the entire treatment period, the likelihood that a good result will be achieved is greater. Giving the patient only enough samples for a day or two while awaiting culture and sensitivity data is a cost-effective way to plan the treatment regimen, but when patients feel better after short-term dosing, the subsequent purchase of the prescription often is not made. Thus, giving samples may have a negative effect among certain populations. And because pharmaceutical companies are under greater pressure to cut costs, distributing samples may become a practice of historical interest only.

Some patients actually cannot afford medication and are at an income level such that other priorities prohibit the purchase of drugs unless symptoms are severe. Health care plans that provide for prescription services certainly encourage greater compliance than plans that do not. Many health providers do not realize that occasionally patients purchase a medication but do not take it, especially if the symptoms subside. If the side effects are too great, the taste or size of the pill is too disagreeable, or the patient's occupation is interfering with compliance, one or more doses of medication may be missed. The longer a prescription drug must be taken, the less likely it is that the dosing period will be completed. It is much easier for a patient to take a medication for 3 days than for 7 days or certainly 14 days. Dosing once a day is always complied with better than dosing three or four times a day, and this fact will probably drive the market place.

Patients can also be noncompliant by failing to notify the physician if symptoms are not improving by a specified time. The failure to follow up with a repeated urinalysis or urine culture might allow an already difficult problem to worsen, complicating the next round of treatment, whether medical or surgical. This noncompliance on the part of the patient can increase costs to the health care system; in the future, it may be necessary for patients to share in this expense when they are noncompliant.

There are other patient-related factors that affect the outcome of the treatment of a urinary tract infection. The patient's own host defense mechanisms play a vital role in the response to treatment. Immunosuppressed patients—such as transplant recipients, patients receiving cancer chemotherapy, or alcoholics—respond more poorly than the normal population. Age, organ failure, and failure on the patient's part to tell the physician about deficiency of glucose 6-phosphate dehydrogenase (G-6-PD) can affect the response to particular antimicrobial agents.

It is very important for the patient to inform the physician of recent previous antimicrobial exposure, which can affect the physician's choice of antibiotic. Prosthetics or foreign bodies in an infected or operative site always increase the possibility of failure of antimicrobial treatment. If a patient has dead or necrotic tissue or pus in the wound without concomitant surgical treatment, the outcome can be jeopardized.

Certain population groups require special attention not only in the treatment of urinary tract infections but also other infectious diseases. Geriatric patients have a higher mortality rate from infections than younger subjects. This may be because of an impaired immune system, the presence of multiple diseases, nutritional factors, or other causes, and certain antibiotics may aggravate pre-existing renal or hepatic impairment (1,2). A deficiency of G-6-PD may result in hemolysis and methemoglobinemia when the erythrocytes are exposed to certain oxidant drugs, such as nitrofurantoin, nalidixic acid, or sulfonamides.

When the presence of anaerobes is suspected because the routine culture is negative, care must be used to obtain and transport the specimen in the proper media; otherwise, the pathogen will not be identified.

It has been this author's experience that patients are neither adequately nor accurately informed by primary care physicians or urologists regarding the true cost and benefit of a urine culture and sensitivity to assure proper selection of an antimicrobial. Given that the true cost to the physician or laboratory in 1995 of performing an accurate urine culture and disk diffusion sensitivity is only about $6 or $7, including technician time, physicians who are operating in a capitated system would probably benefit from performing a culture and sensitivity in their own office in parallel with the treatment selection. For example, if one were to gamble with a complicated infection and provide treatment that costs the patient or the health care system $6/day for 10 days, this $60 could represent savings if a $7 culture and $6/day therapy for 2 days were coupled with another 8 days of $1/day therapy. The total might be half as expensive. If patients and physicians could follow accurate algorithms such as the one in Fig. 1 in a risk-sharing organization, the total health care dollars expended might shrink. In addition, prescribing the most expensive and most powerful broad-spectrum antibiotics often results in increased side effects or development of resistant organisms that can siphon thousands of additional dollars into the health care deficit.

Outcomes Related to the Physician

The principles of antimicrobial therapy are directly related to and must be understood by the physician. If the urologist fails to make the proper diagnosis, a patient's condition can worsen, resulting in hospitalization, sepsis, escalating costs, and, at worst, death. Improper diagnosis can prompt the prescribing of the wrong antimicrobial, which can alter the sensitivity, increase the nosocomial infection rate in a hospital environment, and also cause pressure on the community of resistant organisms. It is hoped that this text thoroughly discusses the decision-making process involved in the selection of a particular drug for urinary tract infection treatment. There are guidelines to follow regarding the initial antibiotic selection before culture and sensitivity data are returned. Then, one must have adequate knowledge to amend the prescription accurately according to the sensitivity and cost-vs.-benefit ratio of the various antimicrobials. If a patient has already been placed on an antibiotic and yet is not responding, i.e., continues to have symptoms, and then comes back into the office for a repeated culture, the caregiver must repeat the culture using antibiotic-removal devices such as β-lactamase (3).

The physician must know the likelihood of an allergic reaction based on the patient's history, type of allergy experienced in the past, and the likelihood of serious allergic reaction to the drug and the cost associated with this untoward consequence. Patients who have experienced a mild reaction to penicillins can usually take cephalosporins without fear of an immediate-type hypersensitivity reaction. These cross-allergenicity reactions should always be taken into consideration in the penicillin- or cephalosporin-allergic population (4). Unfortunately, most physicians are not aware of the many drugs that can aggravate other conditions or diseases that a patient may have or how they can affect other pharmaceutical products that the patient might be taking. For example, how many urologists know or inquire about G-6-PD deficiencies in their patient population or whether the patient is taking H_2 inhibitors or theophylline? All three of these are vitally important factors yet are not routinely queried.

Understanding the principles of antimicrobial therapy requires a thorough knowledge of both drugs and microbes. It not only means that one must be aware that a certain antimicrobial will eradicate *Escherichia coli* 90% of the time in a community and yet only 80% of the time in the hospital; it also requires the ongoing accumulation of data both in the hospital and in the physician's lab regarding resistance percentages in both environments. Sensitivity to all antimicrobials is constantly changing. If physicians are not aware of the change in their particular locale, then they are further increasing the gamble of treatment and the risk of failure, resulting in increased costs of the treatment regimen.

If the physician does sensitivity testing in the office environment, he or she must be aware of the drawback of the disk diffusion test, which is the most commonly used test for detecting microbe susceptibility. The zone sizes for "resistant, intermediate, or susceptible" are based on the average serum concentration and really have very little to do with urine levels of a drug. This test also measures bacteriostatic activity, which could be confusing when bactericidal concentration in the urine is required (5). The disks that test sulfonamides, nalidixic acid, and nitrofurantoin are calibrated for urine levels, however.

The physician often affects the outcome of treatment by prescribing unnecessary antimicrobials. Long-term prophylaxis for surgery has been shown to be ineffective for many years. Even short-term prophylaxis for surgery, in many cases, is now unnecessary because of better surgical techniques and greater sterility. Long-term treatment for UTIs of 10, 14, or 30 days, as has been traditionally employed, is now restricted almost solely to the treatment of true chronic bacterial prostatitis. Even hemorrhagic cystitis is often of viral origin, requiring no antimicrobial treatment at all or limited antimicrobial treatment until the sensitivity is returned. Physicians not uncommonly treat fever of unknown origin on the sole basis of an uncatheterized urine specimen revealing pyuria. By failing to make an accurate diagnosis, they cause resistant bacteria and opportunistic infections, such as candidiasis, to develop in the patient and make it impossible to determine a future urinary diagnosis.

Certain things are essential to understanding antimicrobial principles. As was mentioned previously, the culture and sensitivity are much underutilized tools and should be routinely done in a capitated environment in almost all cases. First, the knowledge that there is no infecting pathogen immediately changes the direction of diagnosis and treatment, which probably results in significant cost savings. However, identification of an organism allows one to select the appropriate antimicrobial. The urologist, having determined where the infection lies, must then make sure that the selected antimicrobial reaches that site. It must not only reach the site but must arrive there in a proper concentration that can be maintained for a significant period of time so as to eradicate the organism through the microbial life cycle. In other words, the chemical must remain at the infected site for a sufficient period of time (which the physician must compute based on the pharmacokinetics of the drug used and the type of organism that is present). Levels of free drug at the site of infection three to five times the minimal inhibitory concentration are recommended to attain the best therapeutic response (5). This information is rarely taught to urology residents today, and this author is amazed at how few practicing urologists, whether neophytes or veterans, possess this knowledge.

The physician is directly responsible for the proper dosing of an antimicrobial and must be aware of the benefits of "bolus" treatment for certain diseases vs. the toxicity of the same. One must not only be aware of, but routinely make use of, the concept of minimal inhibitory concentration (MIC) in selecting the antimicrobial for a particular organism at a particular site of infection. The urologist must know when to change antimicrobials based on culture and sensitivity data or the development of resistance during or after an infection.

All urologists have heard, either from patients or from referring physicians, of a patient with a particular infection taking an antimicrobial for 7 to 10 days without experiencing significant improvement in symptoms, only to be told to take the medication for another 7 to 10 days because the patient "might not have taken the drug long enough." The likelihood of several days of the proper antimicrobial treatment not at least improving symptoms is extremely rare, and yet this practice is common. The timing of treatment is very important and vital to the individual patient's outcome and the outcome of other patients in the community and hospital settings. Too long or too short a duration both can affect bacterial resistance. Therapy for too long contributes significantly to the development of nosocomial infections and toxicity and adverse events in the patient, all of which dramatically increase costs to the health care system.

CONCLUSION

The reader is invited to peruse and study each of the following chapters with the previous comments and principles in mind. More than ever before, urologists now must become expert at diagnosing and treating urinary tract infections not only accurately but efficiently. A failure to acquire these skills will force the payers of health care dollars to look elsewhere for cheaper medicine. Urologists must create the pathways for primary care physicians to follow and serve as consultants on difficult cases.

REFERENCES

1. Guay DRP, Obaid S, Breitenbucher R. Antibiotic use in the elderly. In: Peterson PK, Verhoef J, eds. *The antimicrobial agents annual/2.* Amsterdam: Elsevier; 1987:422–430.
2. Hanno P. Therapeutic principles of antimicrobial therapy and new antimicrobial agents. *Urol Clin North Am* 1986;13:577–590.
3. Sane MA, Mandell GL. Antimicrobial agents, general considerations. In: Gilman AG, Goodman LS, Rall TW, et al., eds. *The pharmacological basis of therapeutics.* New York: Macmillan; 1985:1066–1094.
4. Wilkowske CJ, Hermans PE. General principles of antimicrobial therapy. *Mayo Clin Proc* 1987;62:789.
5. Pratt WB, Fekety R, eds. *Determinants of bacterial response to antimicrobial agents.* New York: Oxford University Press; 1986:3–15.

Antibiotic Therapy in Urology,
edited by S. Grant Mulholland, M.D.,
Lippincott-Raven Publishers, Philadelphia © 1996.

Chapter 2

Antimicrobial Treatment of Pyelonephritis and Sepsis

James A. Roberts

Department of Urology, Tulane Regional Primate Research Center, Covington, Louisiana 70433; and Tulane University School of Medicine, New Orleans, Louisiana 70112

INTRODUCTION

Escherichia coli is by far the most frequent cause of acute pyelonephritis. While therapy of acute pyelonephritis should be designed to eradicate the infection and relieve the symptoms, the prevention of chronic pyelonephritis should also be a goal. Of children and young adults reaching end-stage renal disease, 15–20% do so with a diagnosis of chronic pyelonephritis either with or without vesicoureteral reflux (1). Most of the patients who acquire these renal scars of chronic pyelonephritis have had acute pyelonephritis within the first years of life. Studies in both infants (2) and children (3) have shown that delayed treatment of acute pyelonephritis is probably responsible for the renal scarring and damage associated with chronic pyelonephritis, sometimes called reflux nephropathy. Thus, the prevention of end-stage renal disease from acute pyelonephritis depends both on early diagnosis and rapid and effective treatment to eradicate the bacteria and stop the destructive inflammatory response. When renal damage from this inflammatory response is severe, the remnant kidney is probably insufficient to meet the increased demand on renal function that occurs during the rapid growth of adolescence. It has been hypothesized that this results in both glomerular hyperfiltration and glomerular hypertension in the residual nephrons (4). This, then, would lead to progressive destruction of the remaining nephrons, with focal glomerulosclerosis and further tubular and interstitial disease. The pathogenesis of this end-stage disease may be similar to the progressive chronic renal failure of glomerulonephritis.

Pyelonephritogenic *E. coli* are characterized by the fact that they carry some chromosomally coded factors, such as those for P-fimbriae and type 1 fimbriae, hemolysin production, O and K serotypes, and aerobactin, as well as a less common plasmid-carried gene, colicin V (5). The singular importance of P-fimbriated *E. coli* in the pathogenesis of acute pyelonephritis in humans has been clearly established during the last 10 years in clinical series of both children (6) and adults (7). In addition, a significant positive correlation has been shown between renal dysfunction and receptor density in patients with renal scarring (8). Recent studies have shown that the activation of interleukin-6, which increases in both serum and urine in acute pyelonephritis, appears to depend on adhesion of *E. coli* to urothelial cells, with this cytokine then recruiting polymorphonuclear cells to the site and initiating the inflammatory response (9). This inflammatory response in acute pyelonephritis is known to damage tissue and cause renal damage in experimental models of pyelonephritis. While P-fimbriae are the major single virulence factor that causes adherence to the α-gal-1-4-—gal disaccharide moiety of urothelial glycolipid, these fimbriae have also been found to bind to fibronectin by minor pilar proteins that adhere to urothelial extracellular matrices (10). P-fimbriae therefore are not only responsible for host tropism during development of the infection to produce acute pyelonephritis; once adherent and causing an inflammatory response, binding to fibronectin and exposed cells may be important in the secondary inflammatory response after this epithelial injury. Recent studies of women with acute pyelonephritis have shown an increase in both urinary and serum interleukin-6 and interleukin-8. The association of *E. coli* with hemolysin was found in patients with an increased serum level of interleukin-6. A high concentration of interleukin-8 was found in the urine of patients while affected with acute pyelonephritis; they were later found to have a lowered glomerular filtration rate. This suggests that the renal production of interleukin-8, another inflammatory cytokine, might well be associated with a more intense inflammatory response and thus renal damage in these patients (11). While P-fimbriae appear to be the single most important virulence factor in pyelonephritis (Fig. 1), other adhesins, including the X- and S-fimbriae and afimbrial adhesins, also must be important. Combinations of multiple factors still remain common among strains causing pyelonephritis, particularly those having the combination of P-fimbriae, type 1 fimbriae, hemolysin, and aerobactin. Data on clinical isolates strongly support a clonal hypothesis that certain combinations of virulence factors make a particular bacterial strain more pathogenic (12). Therapy of acute pyelonephritis must be directed at rapid eradication of the *E. coli* causing the disease; in addition, attention must be paid to those patients with bacteremia and sepsis, with consideration for treatment using both antibacterials and agents that counteract the events leading to sepsis.

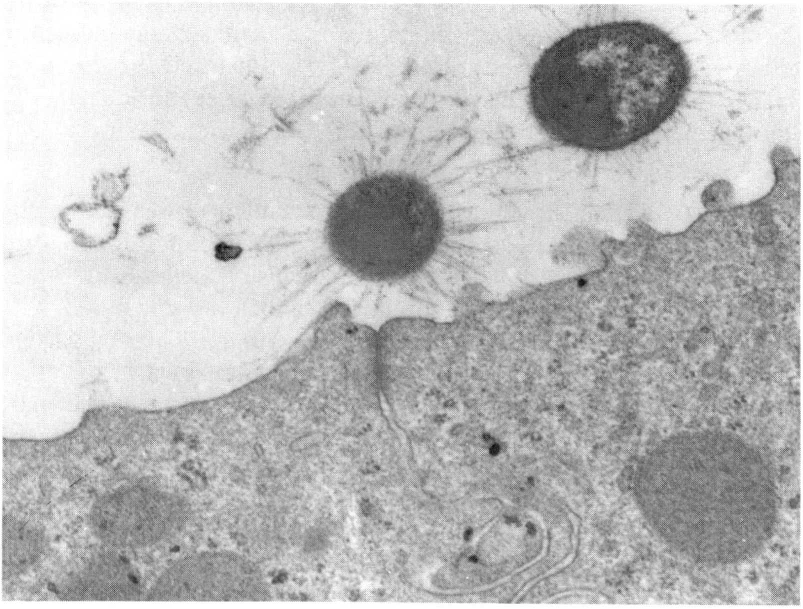

FIG. 1. Transmission electron micrograph showing P-fimbriated *E. coli* adhering to proximal renal tubules in early experimental pyelonephritis in the monkey. ×45000.

ANTIBACTERIAL THERAPY OF ACUTE PYELONEPHRITIS

The ideal drug in the patient with acute pyelonephritis would be one that is bactericidal, shows a broad spectrum, and has a pharmacology that leads to high penetration and concentration in both urine and renal tissue. These drugs include the aminoglycosides, aminopenicillins (amoxicillin or ampicillin, alone or in combination with clavulanic acid or sulbactam), carboxypenicillins (carbenicillin or ticarcillin), uredopenicillins (mezlocillin or piperacillin), monobactams (aztreonam), carbapenems (imipenem or imipenem-cilastatin), cephalosporins, fluoroquinolones, or trimethoprim/ sulfamethoxazole. The ideal drug for acute pyelonephritis may be a fluoroquinolone because of the broad spectrum (except in pregnancy or in childhood). Because of cost, the drugs most frequently used are aminoglycosides, amino or carboxypenicillins, aztreonam, cephalosporins, and fluoroquinolones (13).

A recent methodological review showed that there was only one randomized trial of antibacterial therapy in acute pyelonephritis, and the size of that trial has been questioned. However, the cure rate for usual antibacterial therapy is approximately 90% for either oral or parenteral therapy. This was shown in studies in which certain patients were not included in the evaluation. These usually include children, pregnant women, male patients, the elderly, and patients with diabetes mellitus, an anatomic abnormality such as stones, or azotemia. Under these conditions, the therapy depends on the severity of the illnesses.

The following are combined suggestions of Meyrier and Guibert (13), Pinson et al. (14), Stamm and Hooten (15), Schlager and Lohr (16), and Lucas and Cunningham (17):

1. The young female adult with mild illness and no nausea or vomiting can usually be treated as an outpatient with oral antibiotics for 10 to 14 days, these most frequently being trimethoprim/sulfamethoxazole or any fluoroquinolone. A new oral drug, loracarbef, as compared with cephalosporin or floxacin appears to be efficacious in eradicating uncomplicated pyelonephritis when the patient has mild disease (18).

2. Female adults with severe infection or possible sepsis as shown by systemic symptoms, high fever, and nausea and vomiting can usually be hospitalized and parenteral therapy administered until the fever is gone. Therapy in this cause would be either trimethoprim/sulfamethoxazole, ceftriaxone, ciprofloxacin, ofloxacin, or gentamycin (with or without ampicillin), all given parenterally until the patient is afebrile, when oral drugs may be continued for a total treatment of 10 to 14 days. Cefetamet pivoxil appears to have effects comparable with those of cefadroxil (19), as also does netilmicin, a new aminoglycoside, as found by studies in both children (20) and adults (21). Whether coverage for gram-positive organisms such as enterococci is needed would depend on the frequency of these organisms in the community or hospital as well as the result of the Gram's stain of the organisms in the urine.

In patients with acute pyelonephritis and sepsis syndrome, symptoms should resolve rapidly (within 48 to 72 hours). If not, further evaluation should be done, including renal ultrasonography, plain x-ray of the abdomen, or intravenous pyelogram. Many, however, do a renal ultrasonogram within 24 to 48 hours of admission to rule out ureteral obstruction. In some patients, computerized tomography (CT) of the kidney is necessary to determine the extent of the disease and, if the patient is not responding to treatment, the possibility of the presence of perinephric or renal abscess.

3. Pregnant women should be closely monitored for asymptomatic bacteriuria, and if found the bacteriuria should be treated to prevent acute pyelonephritis. Nitrofurantoin appears to be the drug of choice because of its high concentration in the urine but low levels in the maternal serum as well as in the fetus. The addition of clavulanic acid to ampicillin has improved its efficacy and, though not well studied in pregnancy, there is no contraindication to its use during pregnancy (17). Hospitalization is recommended for the therapy of acute pyelonephritis in pregnant patients because of the small percentage (2%) who develop acute respiratory distress

syndrome after the initiation of antibacterial therapy (22). The drugs suggested for therapy during acute pyelonephritis in pregnancy include a cephalosporin (cephalexin), gentamycin (with or without ampicillin), aztreonam, and trimethoprim/sulfamethoxazole (except in the last trimester).

Sulfonamides confer some risk of hyperbilirubinemia if given near delivery. The combination with trimethoprim (trimethoprim/sulfamethoxazole) enhances the efficacy of the sulfonamide alone, but since it acts to inhibit dihydrofolate reductase, it could create a hazard for the fetus. The best course of action is not to use this drug in the last trimester. The fluoroquinolones are also avoided because of the question of their effects on growing bone (17).

4. In neonates it is suggested that broad coverage for both group B streptococci and Enterobacteriaceae is necessary (16). This most frequently includes ampicillin with the addition of trimethoprim/ sulfamethoxazole or a broad-spectrum cephalosporin. If symptoms are severe, gentamycin is also added to therapy.

5. In complicated infections (diabetes, stone, and others) with severe illness (bacteremia and sepsis), any obstruction must be relieved, and initial therapy should probably consist of parenteral fluoroquinolones, or, if the patient is not allergic to penicillin, imipenem/cilastatin, or ticarcillin/clavulanate, although third-generation cephalosporins such as ceftazidime or ceftriaxone are also used. Antibiotic therapy is summarized in Table 1.

COMPLICATING FACTORS

Pyonephrosis

This is a serious complication of infection with ureteral obstruction. Pyonephrosis most simply is defined as purulent material in an obstructed collecting system, being obtained by either ureteral catheter or percutaneous access. When the infected renal pelvis and calyces develop invasive disease, this becomes acute pyelonephritis, and in the presence of continued obstruction renal function rapidly deteriorates and sepsis ensues. This has often been associated with staghorn calculi, which become obstructing and in the past have often been treated by nephrectomy. With the advent of percutaneous access and treatment of such stones, percutaneous access of a pyelonephritic kidney with ureteral obstruction in combination with antibacterial therapy is then followed by treatment of the offending obstruction. In these cases, most kidneys have been salvaged. Indeed, in a recent review of 23 cases of pyonephrosis, nephrectomy was needed in only 5 patients after relief of the obstruction. Definitive therapy of the obstructive disorder included percutaneous nephrolithotomy, ureteroscopic

TABLE 1. *Treatment of acute pyelonephritis (APN)*

Condition	Parenteral	Oral
Female adults		
Mild APN		Trimethoprim/ sulfamethoxazole Amoxicillin w. clavulanate Ciprofloxacin Ofloxacin Norfloxacin
APN with sepsis	Trimethoprim/ sulfamethoxazole Gentamicin w. ampicillin Amoxicillin w. sulbactam Ceftazidime Ceftriaxone Ciprofloxacin Ofloxacin	
Complicated APN with sepsis	*Relieve any ureteral obstruction* Ciprofloxacin Ofloxacin Imipenem/cilastatin Ticarcillin/clavulanate Piperacillin	
Pregnant women		
Asymptomatic bacteriuria		Nitrofurantoin macrocrystals or Macrobid Cephalexin Amoxicillin w. clavulanate
APN	Trimethoprim/ sulfamethoxazole Cefazolin Ceftazidime Ceftriaxone Gentamicin w. ampicillin Aztreonam	
Children		
Neonatal APN	Ampicillin Cefazolin If severe, add gentamicin	
Infant APN	Ampicillin Cefazolin Ceftazidime If severe, add gentamicin	

treatment of ureteral calculi, and extracorporeal shock wave lithotripsy of obstructing stones (23).

Emphysematous Pyelonephritis

This form of acute pyelonephritis is associated with the production of gas within the renal parenchyma. This gas may further extend into the perinephric space. It is often associated with ureteral obstruction and uncontrolled diabetes mellitus and is believed to be caused by renal ischemia occurring during acute pyelonephritis, resulting in a low oxygen tension and thereby producing anaerobic metabolism. Enterobacteriaceae, being facultative anaerobes, are able to ferment glucose to lactate and carbon dioxide. It has thus been suggested that carbon dioxide is the gas responsible for the appearance on x-ray. Nephrectomy has been the treatment of choice in the past because even with immediate nephrectomy, studies reported in 1985 a mortality rate of 42% (24). Abdominal CT is an additional modality for the diagnosis, although it is usually apparent on a plain x-ray film of the abdomen (25). A recent report showed that a combination of percutaneous management and antibiotics in cases of emphysematous pyelonephritis associated with obstruction was successful (26). Thus, in the patient with obstruction who is too ill for surgery, percutaneous drainage and antibiotics should be considered. In the absence of obstruction, nephrectomy would still be indicated in these patients to control both their diabetes and the infection.

Xanthogranulomatous Pyelonephritis

This destructive form of acute pyelonephritis is usually associated with stones, most frequently staghorn calculi. It is believed that the pathologic appearance of the kidney is caused by a chronic inflammatory response to bacteria that have not been totally eradicated because of insufficient antibacterial therapy. The patients usually present with superimposed acute pyelonephritis with or without pyonephrosis and a nonfunctioning kidney, which is treated with antibacterials and nephrectomy.

PATHOGENESIS OF SEPSIS FROM ACUTE PYELONEPHRITIS

Sepsis has been reported to be the 13th leading cause of death in the United States for people over 1 year of age. It has a mortality rate of 40% if septic shock occurs. Though antibacterial therapy may effectively treat the acute pyelonephritis, this does not necessarily reverse the host response to infection (27).

In Vitro Study of Endotoxin

In an in vitro study on endotoxin release from bacteria, endotoxin release was varied but reproducible for each species of bacteria studied. It is thought that the release of endotoxin is in part caused by the rapidity

TABLE 2. *In vitro study of endotoxin*

Bacteria	Antibacterial causing least release of endotoxin
Escherichia coli	Gentamicin
	Imipenem
	Fluoroquinolone
Pseudomonas aeruginosa	Ceftazidime
	Imipenem
Klebsiella pneumoniae	Imipenem

of bacterial killing, and that those antibacterials that kill the bacteria rapidly cause less bacterial endotoxin release. The correlation between rapidity of bacterial killing and endotoxin release is not perfect, however, as ceftazidime kills bacteria rapidly but fails to inhibit endotoxin release, while the quinolones, which also kill bacteria rapidly, show good inhibition of endotoxin release of both *E. coli* and *Klebsiella pneumoniae* but not *Pseudomonas*. These in vitro data would suggest that imipenem and the quinolones would have the advantage of rapid bacterial killing and lowest release of endotoxin. It may be that endotoxin plays a larger role in the morbidity that occurs during antibiotic treatment than originally thought. The antibacterials associated with the lowest rates of release of endotoxin from the bacteria studied is shown in Table 2 (28).

Sepsis Syndrome

While the release of endotoxin during antibacterial therapy must be considered, mechanisms to prevent the effect of the release of endotoxin and modulate the response of the host are necessary. Many names have been used to describe the condition of the patient with sepsis. These include bacteremia, sepsis, systemic inflammatory response syndrome (SIRS), and septic shock (29). As previously noted, once shock occurs, the mortality rate is greater than 40% despite therapy. It is now obvious from studies in the past 10 years that septic shock is the result of endogenous protein and phospholipid mediators being secreted by the injured host, eventually leading to the release of nitric oxide, which produces profound cardiovascular effects and shock (30). While the clinical pattern of hemodynamic and metabolic derangements that occur with gram-negative infection is present in septic shock, an identical syndrome can occur with trauma and tissue injury, pancreatitis, and the ischemia associated with hemorrhagic shock. The pathophysiologic events that occur result in multiple organ dysfunction and death. It is now known that the lipid A protein of endotoxin (lipopolysaccharide) is the most important initiating factor of sepsis. Because of this, polyclonal and monoclonal antibody preparations to the lipid A of endotoxin have been developed and tested in clinical trials (31). While some of these trials have had a positive result, others have not (32). It is felt that the therapeutic benefit may be limited to only a subset of patients and that early diagnosis of gram-negative infection in patients with sepsis would be necessary to begin effective treatment. As an example, while experimental therapy with corticosteroids is successful in moderating sepsis and preventing shock and death in bacterial meningitis, it is effective only if treatment is begun early (33). In bacterial meningitis, high endotoxin levels produce high levels of tumor necrosis factor within the meninges, which is associated with a higher morbidity rate. Because of this, treatment of patients having meningitis with corticosteroids to decrease the inflammatory response and cytokine activity is now done prior to the initiation of antibacterial therapy, which appears to cause more endotoxin release.

More recent studies concentrate on the early events that occur following the release of lipopolysaccharide (LPS) from bacteria. Two events occur: First, neutrophils release a bactericidal/permeability-increasing protein (BPI), which binds LPS and prevents macrophage activation and has been shown to be protective against otherwise lethal endotoxemia in rodents. The release of this compound, therefore, leads to modulation of the effects of lipopolysaccharide release. Second, a lipopolysaccharide-binding protein (LBP) (a compound normally present in human serum) increases over 100-fold during the acute phase response because of infectious activation of interleukin-6. The LBP binds to the lipid moiety LPS, forming an LPS-LBP complex. This complex interacts with its receptor (CD14) on monocytes, macrophages, and neutrophils, and genes encoding the production of cytokines are thus induced (27). While the release of interleukin-6 leads to the acute-phase response, interleukin-6 is not thought to be damaging to the host. However, the release of interleukin-1 and tumor necrosis factor were shown to be important in a model of overwhelming bacterial sepsis in baboons (34). Tumor necrosis factor concentration in serum peaked rapidly and was followed by increase in interleukin-1b and gamma interferon. Immunization against tumor necrosis factor prevented death. All animals not passively immunized in this manner developed shock, multiple organ dysfunction, and death (35). Similar experiments in the rhesus monkey have shown rapid induction of interleukin-6 and tumor necrosis factor, and in those animals that died of sepsis as opposed to those who survived, a continuing increase in serum concentration of both interleukin-6 and tumor necrosis factor occurred (36) (Fig. 2).

Much experimental activity is now ongoing in an attempt to block the cytokine cascade and prevent the events leading to septic death. Since tumor necrosis factor appears to be the earlier mediator of septic shock,

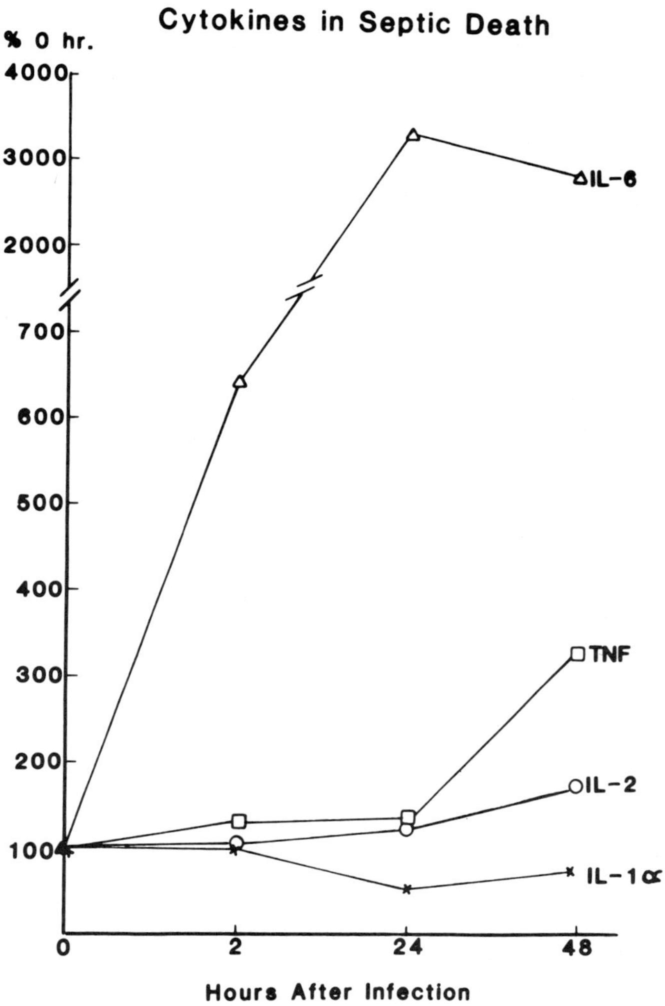

FIG. 2. The cytokine response in sera of monkeys that died of sepsis from experimental pyelonephritis. Note the marked rise in interleukin-6 and continuing rise in tumor necrosis factor until death at 48 hours after untreated infection was induced. From Roberts et al., ref. 36.

treatment with antitumor necrosis factor antibodies is now being studied in human trials (37). Although interleukin-1 by itself does not produce death in animals (as tumor necrosis factor does), an interleukin-1 antagonist has reduced mortality rates in animal models and is now in phase 2 trials in humans (38). Other mediators now being considered are surface adhesion molecules of both endothelial cells and neutrophils, including CD11/18 and CD14. These appear to be direct mediators of the derangement seen in septic shock, and blocking their actions might be another effective method of preventing or attenuating shock using monoclonal antibodies to these receptors. Tissue injury occurring during ischemia from acute pyelonephritis has been suggested to be one cause of renal damage in experimental models, the damage being caused by release of toxic forms of oxygen during the respiratory burst of phagocytosis or during reperfusion. Allopurinol, which prevents the formation of these toxic forms of oxygen because of its activity as a xanthine oxidase inhibitor during reperfusion, does prevent the reperfusion injury (39). Endothelium-dependent vascular relaxation has been found to be caused by nitric oxide, which after activation by toxic forms of oxygen appears to be the endogenous activator of soluble guanylate cyclase. The increase in cyclic guanosine monophosphate (cGMP) that ensues causes nitric oxide-induced vasodilation, which may lead to shock, changes in leukocyte adhesion, and modulation of certain types of neurotransmission (40). Since this seems to be the cause of the vascular effects during sepsis, one trial has been begun using a nitric oxide synthase inhibitor, with some early encouraging results (41). In addition to the above, endotoxin causes release of platelet-activating factor (PAF) from macrophages, polymorphonuclear cells, platelets, and endothelial cells. This potent inflammatory mediator increases cell adhesion and activates endothelial cells by the formation of toxic oxygen species and arachidonic acid metabolites. Indeed, clinical trials of PAF antagonists and septic shock are now under way. It is probable that ongoing clinical trials will lead to suggestions for therapy in different patient populations at different stages of the sepsis syndrome and inflammatory response; therapy will probably be a combination of antibacterials and monoclonal antibodies to cytokines, particularly tumor necrosis factor, as well as soluble receptors to combine with these cytokines.

BACTERIAL RESISTANCE

Despite the synthesis of many antibacterials over the last 30 years, we have reached a crisis in the developement of antibacterial resistance. As stated in the recent review by Neu (42), despite all these antibiotics, a person could die in a hospital in New York, San Francisco, Paris, Barcelona, Tokyo, or Singapore as a result of a resistant bacterial infection. This resistance may occur as a result of chromosomal changes or by the exchange of genetic material by plasmids or transposons. It is thought that this increasing resistance is the consequence of the extensive, uncontrolled use of antibiotics both in hospitals and the community. The hospital and nursing home setting is ideal for the transfer of bacterial resistance, producing resident resistant strains that create difficult-to-treat nosocomial infections. While not a frequent cause of

TABLE 3. *Emerging bacterial resistance in urinary tract pathogens*

Bacteria	Antibiotics to which developing resistance
E. coli	β-lactams (amoxicillin, ampicillin/clavulanate, and sulbactam) Trimethoprim/sulfamethoxazole
Enterobacter	β-lactams (cephalosporins, penicillins, ampicillin/clavulanate)
Pseudomonas	β-lactams (penicillins, cephalosporins, monobactams) Aminoglycosides Carbapenems Fluoroquinolones
Enterococci	β-lactams (penicillins, cephalosporins, monobactams) Carbapenems Fluoroquinolones Vancomycin
Serratia	β-lactams (cephalosporins) Fluoroquinolones Aminoglycosides Trimethoprim/sulfamethoxazole
Klebsiella	β-lactams (cephalosporins, monobactams) Aminoglycosides

From Neu, ref. 42.

acute pyelonephritis, *Staphylococcus aureus* is the most frightening example, as in excess of 95% of all *S. aureus* is resistant to penicillin, ampicillin, and the newer antipseudomonas penicillins.

E. coli remains the most common cause of acute pyelonephritis in the normal urinary tract. At present 30% of community-acquired and up to 50% of hospital-acquired urinary tract infections are resistant to amoxicillin, whether used alone or in combination with the β-lactam inhibitor clavulanate or sulbactam. The cheapest and at one time most effective antibacterial in the treatment of urinary tract infecions, trimethoprim/sulfamethoxazole, is now ineffective because of bacterial resistance in *E. coli* (Table 3).

Enterobacter species and *Pseudomonas* species, after *E. coli* the most common causes of nosocomial urinary tract infections, now show an increasing incidence of resistance to β-lactams (including third-generation cephalosporins and antipseudomonal penicillins), aminoglycosides, carbapenems, and fluoroquinolones.

While an infrequent cause of urinary tract infections in most settings, enterococci are now becoming a more serious problem, with the early development of resistance to β-lactams, particularly the penicillins, to the carbapenem imipenem, even in combination with cilastatin, to the macrolides, fluoroquinolones, and now the last effective drug, vancomycin.

Mechanisms to decrease the emergence of resistant strains should include simple hygienic practices, such as hand washing between patient contacts, the use of the simplest antibacterial rather than the newest broad-spectrum fluoroquinolone in uncomplicated acute cystitis, and the use of short-term prophylactic antibiotics when indicated. We as physicians are responsible for following these simple tenets, and the pharmaceutical industry should not promote their newest antibacterial inappropriately.

REFERENCES

1. Roberts JA. Etiology and pathophysiology of pyelonephritis. *Am J Kidney Dis* 1991;17:1–9.
2. Winberg J, Bollgren I, Kallenius G, Mollby R, Svenson SB. Clinical pyelonephritis and focal renal scarring. A selected review of pathogenesis, prevention, and prognosis. *Pediatr Clin North Am* 1982;29:801–813.
3. Winter AL, Hardy BE, Alton DJ, Arubs GS, Churchill BM. Acquired renal scars in children. *J Urol* 1983;129:1190–1194.
4. Brenner BM. Hemodynamically mediated glomerular injury and the progressive nature of kidney disease. *Kidney Int* 1983;23:647–655.
5. Johnson JR. Virulence factoirs in Escherichia coli urinary tract infection. *Clin Microbiol Rev* 1991;4:80–128.
6. Elo J, Tallgren LG, Vaisanen V, Korhonen SB, Makela PH. Association of P and other fimbriae with clinical pyelonephritis in children. *Scand J Urol Nephrol* 1985;19:281–284.
7. Latham R, Stamm W. Role of fimbriated Escherichia coli in urinary tract infections in adult women: correlation with localization studies. *J Infect Dis* 1984;149:835–840.
8. Svenson SB, Kallenius G. Density and localization of P-fimbriae-specific receptors of mammalian cells: fluorescence-activated cell analysis. *Infection* 1983;1:6–12.
9. Hedges S, Agace W, Svensson M, Sjögren A, Ceska M, Svanborg C. Urothelial cells are part of a mucosal cytokine network. *Infect Immun* 1994;62:2315–2321.
10. Westerlund B, Van Die I, Hoekstra W, Virkola R, Korhonen TK. P fimbriae of uropathogenic Escherichia coli as multifunctional adherence organelles. *Zbl Bakt* 1993;278:229–237.
11. Jacobson SH, Hylander B, Wretlind B, Brauner A. Interleukin-6 and interleukin-8 in serum and urine in patients with acute pyelonephritis in relation to bacterial-virulence-associated traits and renal function. *Nephron* 1994;67:172–179.
12. Achtman M, Pluschke G. Clonal analysis of descent and virulence among sected Escherichia coli. *Annu Rev Microbiol* 1986;40:184–210.
13. Meyrier A, Guibert J. Diagnosis and drug treatment of acute pyelonephritis. *Drugs* 1992;44:356–367.
14. Pinson AG, Philbrick JT, Lindbeck GH, Schorling JB. Oral antibiotic therapy for acute pyelonephritis. *J Gen Intern Med* 1992;7:544–553.
15. Stamm WE, Hooten TM. Mangement of urinary tract infections in adults. *N Engl J Med* 1993;329:1328–1334.
16. Schlager TA, Lohr JA. Urinary tract infection in outpatient febrile infants and children younger than 5 years of age. *Pediatr Ann* 1993;22:505–509.
17. Lucas MJ, Cunningham FG. Urinary infection in pregnancy. *Clin Obstet Gynecol* 1993;36:855–868.
18. Hyslop DL, Bischoff W. Loracarbef (LY163892) versus cefaclor and norfloxacin in the treatment of uncomplicated pyelonephritis. *Am J Med* 1992;92 (suppl 6A):6A86S–6A94S).
19. Stathakis C, Roulleau N, Libert M, Germano G, Kissling M. Cefetamet pivoxil in acute pyelonephritis: an open study. *Curr Med Res Opin* 1990;12:43–50.
20. Vigano A, Principi N, Brivio L, Tommasi P, Stasi P, Villa AD. Comparison of 55 milligrams of netilmicin per kilogram of body weight once daily versus 2 milligrams per kilogram thrice daily for treatment of gram-negative pyelonephritis in children. *Antimicrob Agents Chemother* 1992;36:1499–1503.
21. Bailey RR, Lynn KL, Robson RA, Peddie BA, Smith A. Comparison of ciprofloxacin with netilmicin for the treatment of acute pyelonephritis. *NZ Med J* 1992;105:102–103.

22. Cunningham, FG, Lucas ML, Hankins GDV. Pulmonary injury complicating antepartum pyelonephritis. *Am J Obstet Gynecol* 1987;156:797–807.
23. Shahatto N, Al Awadhi NA, Ghazali S. Emphysematous pyelonephritis: surgical implications. *Br J Urol* 1990;66:572–574.
24. Ahlering TE, Boyd SD, Hamilton CL. Emphysematous pyelonephritis—a 5 year experience with 13 patients. *J Urol* 1985;134:1086–1088.
25. Bohlman ME, Sweren BS, Khazan R, Minkin SD, Goldman SM, Fishman EK. Emphysematous pyelitis and emphysematous pyelonephritis characterized by computerized tomography. *South Med J* 1991;84:1438–1443.
26. Koh KBH, Lam HS, Lee SH. Emphysematous pyelonephritis: drainage or nephrectomy? *Br J Urol* 1993;71:609–611.
27. Darville T, Girior B, Jacobs R. The systemic inflammatory response syndrome (SIRS): immunology and potential immunotherapy. *Infection* 1993;21:279–290.
28. Eng RHK, Smith SM, Fan-Havard P, Ogbara T. Effects of antibiotics on endotoxin release from gram-negative bacteria. *Diagn Microbiol Infect Dis* 1993;16:185–189.
29. Darville T, Giroir B, Jacobs R. The systemic inflammatory response syndrome (SIRS): immunology and potential immunotherapy. *Infection* 1993;21:279–289.
30. Dunn DL. Gram-negative bacterial sepsis and sepsis syndrome. *Surg Clin North Am* 1994;74:621–635.
31. Ulevitch RJ. Recognition of bacterial endotoxins by receptor-dependent mechanisms. *Adv Immunol* 1993;53:267–289.
32. Chmiel H. Overview of the management of sepsis. *Clin Infect Dis* 1993;17 (suppl 2):S525–S526.
33. Odio CM, Faingezicht I, Paris M, Nassar M, Baltodano A, Rogers J, Sβez-Llorens X, Olsen KD, McCracken GH. The beneficial effects or early dexamethasone administration in infants and children with bacterial meningitis. *N Engl J Med* 1991;324:1525–1531.
34. Hesse DG, Tracey KJ, Fong Y, et al. Cytokine appearance in human endotoxemia and primate bacteremia. *Surg Gynecol Obstet* 1988;166:147–153.
35. Fischer E, Marano MA, Van Zee KJ, et al. Interleukin-1 receptor blockade improves survival and hemodynamic performance in Escherichia coli septic shock, but fails to alter host responses to sublethal endotoxemia. *J Clin Invest* 1992;89:1551–1557.
36. Roberts JA, Kaack MB, Baskin G, Martin LN. Events leading to septic death from experimental acute pyelonephritis in the monkey. *J Urol* 1993;150:1030–1033.
37. Pennington JE. Therapy with antibody to tumor necrosis factor in sepsis. *Clin Infect Dis* 1993;17 (suppl 2):S515–519.
38. Fisher CJ, Dhainaut J-F, Opal SM, et al. Recombinant human interleukin 1 receptor antagonist in the treatment of patients with sepsis syndrome. Results from a randomized, double-blind, placebo-controlled trial. *JAMA* 1994;271:1836–1848.
39. Roberts JA, Kaack MB, Baskin G. Treatment of experimental pyelonephritis in the monkey. *J Urol* 1990;143:150–154.
40. Van Dervort AL, Yan L, Madara PJ, et al. Nitric oxide regulates endotoxin-inducerd TNF—a production by human neutrophils. *J Immunol* 1994;152:4102–4109.
41. Geroulanos S, Schilling J, Cakmakei M, Jung HH, Lariader F. Inhibition of NO synthesis in septic shock. *Lancet* 1992;339:435.
42. Neu HC. The crisis in antibiotic resistance. *Science* 1992;257:1064–1073.

Antibiotic Therapy in Urology,
edited by S. Grant Mulholland, M.D.,
Lippincott-Raven Publishers, Philadelphia © 1996.

Chapter 3

Treatment of Complicated and Uncomplicated Urinary Tract Infections

Rodney U. Anderson

Department of Urology, Stanford University School of Medicine and Santa Clara Valley Medical Center, San Jose, California 95128

If the tables of contents of current journals are any indication, there appears to be less clinical interest these days in the medical problem of urinary tract infections (UTI). Despite this lack of coverage and seeming dearth of investigative endeavor, uncomplicated and complicated urinary tract infections continue to occupy a large portion of the primary care physician's and urologist's practice. Many individuals suffer symptoms and morbidity of such infections, causing us to spend enormous amounts of our health care dollars on antimicrobial treatments and hospitalization; additionally, we suffer economic loss from lost work time. In extreme situations, some unfortunate individuals with poor host resistance factors encounter virulent organisms and lose their lives. There were over 6 million office visits for UTI tracked in 1991 (1). UTI continues to be a leading cause of gram-negative sepsis in hospitalized patients, and catheter-associated infections are thought to raise mortality rates as an independent risk factor by about 14% (2). It is easy to become complacent about the problem of urinary tract infections because we harbor the illusion that we are invincible with our armamentarium of antibiotic formulations. While it is true that we are much better prepared to deal with a serious UTI, we should not be complacent about the insidious development of antimicrobial resistance factors and patterns that may cause the problem to pop up and bite us when we least expect it.

This chapter addresses in a general way the concept of uncomplicated vs. complicated infections. Other chapters in the book focus on and amplify these themes. General categories of infection include uncomplicated UTI in young (premenopausal) women, recurrent infection in young women, uncomplicated pyelonephritis in young women, complicated infection in all adults, and asymptomatic bacteriuria in all adults.

CLINICAL PRESENTATION

The simplest uncomplicated infection is bacterial cystitis, defined as pain on micturition, urinary frequency or a sense of residual urine, pyuria of at least 10 leukocytes per high power microscopic field (HPF), and bacteriuria of at least 10^3 colony-forming units (CFU) per milliliter of urine (3). This definition does not mean that one should exclude from this diagnostic category those individuals with signs and symptoms of UTI without painful micturition. Many women suffer only a sense of discomfort or slight urgency with significant bacteriuria and pyuria. Bacteriuria in the absence of pyuria may represent colonization of the urinary tract rather than infection, yet it remains another category of UTI that begs refinement into complicated or uncomplicated; it is certainly complicated if you try to eradicate the clinical condition in an elderly individual who may suffer significant adverse effects from powerful antimicrobial agents (4). As will be appreciated by perusing the various approaches to complicated infections set forth by the authors in this textbook, careful consideration needs to be given to the clinical factors of age, host condition, infecting organism, and host response.

Clinical cure is determined when all clinical signs and symptoms subside during treatment, no clinical evidence of infection exists at the time the drug is discontinued, and urine cultures taken during and 1 week after discontinuation of treatment remain negative. It is not unusual, however, to have that same patient back in the clinic or office with yet another symptomatic urinary tract infection within 1 to 3 months of that clinical cure. The patient must now be characterized as suffering from recurrent UTI if noncompliance, poor antimicrobial absorption, resistant organisms, or the presence of a structural abnormality, making it a complicated infection, has been ruled out as a cause of recurrence. The young woman thus deserves placement into the category of recurrent bacteriuria and represents an entirely different problem. About 20% of first-time urinary tract infections in young, premenopausal women fall into this characteristic pattern, thought to be the consequence of a genetic predispostion as described below.

CHARACTERIZATION OF COMPLICATED INFECTIONS

It is traditional to divide urinary tract infections into complicated and uncomplicated groups; this division of diagnosis may suggest a more extensive treatment program for the complicated patients. The literature proposes the definition of a complicated infection to imply an abnormal host factor. If the host, or patient, has some anatomic, immunologic, or metabolic abnormality, the urinary tract infection in that setting should be considered as complicated. Most commonly patients who have diabetes, stones, or anatomic abnormalities, who have been immunocompromised, who are pregnant, who have neurogenic bladder, or who are elderly are those defined as having complicated infections. An uncomplicated urinary tract infection can be serious, however. If one adheres to the traditional connotation that a complicated infection requires an abnormality of the host, then some serious urinary tract infections, including urosepsis and even abscess formation, are not technically complicated. And yet the clinical management of these patients is not simple. It is true, of course, that most serious urinary tract infections with invasion occur in individuals who have some compromise of their natural resistance—age, immunologic compromise, diabetes, or pregnancy. Does the otherwise healthy individual who develops an acute urinary tract infection after being catheterized for a residual urine in the doctor's office qualify as a case of complicated urinary tract infection?

I believe most physicians would agree that recurrent urinary tract infection in an otherwise healthy young woman represents a complicated infection although the host is otherwise healthy. One could state that any urinary tract infection that does not demonstrate an expected biologic response of eradication and elimination of symptoms becomes complicated, requiring further work-up and analysis if not further, and perhaps more powerful, antimicrobial agents.

One cannot simply extrapolate experience in treating uncomplicated infections to complicated ones. The organisms are usually different, and naturally the host is altered in some way that affects response to therapy. There have not been controlled trials of treatment regimens in these individuals, and hence a lot of individual assessment is required.

Many of our traditional clinical trial reports for new drug applications are defined as randomized comparisons of agents used in treatment of complicated urinary tract infections. Careful study of the patients and methods used, however, reveals that many of these cases are not truly complicated, and some cases are clearly less complicated than others. Usually, two equivalent agents are compared and the outcome shows no difference in clinical and microbiologic assessment—implying that the new agent is as effective as the old standard, often with less frequent dosing and consequently less cost; similarly, many times the new agent performs equally well with less adverse reactions.

Characterization of Risk Factors

We characterize patients as falling into a complicated or uncomplicated status with their current UTI. The previous methodology involved defining an infection as complicated based on some abnormality or location of the infection anatomically. A more rational approach is to evaluate each patient individually and characterize all the risk factors before assigning the label complicated. The mere presence of a stone in the urinary tract does not necessarily make that individual infection a complicated one; it depends on where the stone is located, whether it has struvite chemical composition and bacteria in its interstices, and whether it is obstructive and playing a major role in the morbidity of the infection.

In addition to a compromised host, risk factors for complication also include demographic features, such as the patient's socioeconomic status, whether the infection was acquired during hospitalization, and what kind of organism and resistance pattern are involved. Also relevant is what kind of urinary tract infection this otherwise healthy individual may have had—previous infections during the year and what microbiologic response occurred during the last treatment. Has there been recent use of antibiotics? Even external risk factors such as the use of birth control devices (diaphragms and condoms) may be involved in the development of infection. Progestational agents may be important. We probably should stratify female patients for treatment based on how close they are to menopause.

Factors that lend themselves to creating complicated UTI include intrinsic anatomic features such as urinary tract obstruction, stasis, and vesicoureteral reflux. Pregnancy and old age are natural biologic developments that make management of bacteriuria problematic. We now understand that genetic factors and expression of genes make a difference in the propensity to become colonized with virulent organisms. Women with Lewis blood-group nonsecretor and recessive phenotypes and biologic differences in bladder and kidney host cell receptor sites are examples. Extrinsic factors such as instrumentation of the urinary tract have caused significant infections for hundreds of years. The modern indwelling catheter represents one of the leading iatrogenic causes of nosocomial urinary tract infections and clearly is a causal factor in many unnecessary cases of fatal gram-negative sepsis in hospitals.

What determines whether or not a patient becomes bacteremic? Virtually all patients who die of urinary tract infection are bacteremic (5). Bacteremia does not appear to be related to development of resistance in strains of typical *Escherichia coli* (6).

The spectrum of causative agents in complicated infections is different. These organisms, unlike the narrow and predictable spectrum in uncomplicated infection, may be resistant to multiple antimicrobial agents. Culture of the urine makes up the foundation of management in this setting. It is difficult to generalize about management. For empiric therapy, the fluoroquinolones probably represent the best outpatient treatment, providing a broad spectrum of antimicrobial activity and achieving high levels of drug concentration in the urine and associated tissues.

Once these characteristics of the patient and the infection are established, the physician is able to follow more standardized clinical pathways and perhaps treat variable UTIs with different antimicrobial agents and for different lengths of time. Each subcategory of patients should be treated in a slightly different fashion.

Infections in Male Patients

It has always been problematic to categorize urinary tract infections in male patients, and as a matter of fact they have usually been considered complicated because they represent involvement of the ancillary genital prostate gland and its enlargement with age. One considers residual urine and poor bladder emptying to contribute to this complicated infection. Are all urinary tract infections in male patients complicated? Do they warrant an expensive work-up? There is no compelling evidence to suggest that benign prostatic hypertrophy and consequent outlet obstruction and residual urine is responsible for an increased incidence of UTI in the older age group. Post-void residual (PVR) urine volumes are not statistically significant. Male patients can have uncomplicated, simple cystitis, usually from sexual intercourse, either vaginal or rectal.

Appropriate workup of UTI in men should include a good genitourologic history, physical exam, and routine blood tests. Urodynamic studies should include a uroflow and PVR determination by ultrasound. An ultrasonogram of kidneys, bladder, and prostate should be followed by an intravenous urogram for any discovered abnormalities. Cystoscopy should be performed only if there is some clinical indication. A semen culture is not as good as an accurate segmented localization study (4-glass) to rule out prostatitis.

Even if we categorize simple infections in men as uncomplicated, the treatment outcomes in men are usually less satisfactory than in women with regard to both clinical and microbiologic testing. Much of this refractory treatment outcome as opposed to pathophysiology can be explained on the basis of age, obstruction, and anatomic abnormality in men. There are also variations in the type of organism seen in men vs. women, more *Staphylococcus* species, *Enterobacter*, *Serratia*, and *Pseudomonas* in men and more *E. coli* and *Klebsiella* seen in women. The MIC levels for men are also usually higher (7).

PATHOPHYSIOLOGY: VIRULENCE OF ORGANISMS AND BACTERIAL ATTACHMENT

The natural history of acute uncomplicated UTI includes the factor of colonization in the vagina and eventually into the urethra. Some female patients by virtue of a genetic predisposition become carriers of organisms in the vagina. It is thought that sexual intercourse is the mechanical factor most associated with seeding the urinary tract.

Most bacteria that contaminate the urinary tract are repelled by acidity, hypo-osmolality, the glycosamine mucoid layer of the urinary tract, and leukocyte mobilization. Some organisms are able to initiate infections by adhering to the urothelium. This adherence property appears to be accommodated by fundamental biologic differences that are genetically expressed by individuals. Schaeffer et al. (8) have shown that there is considerable evidence for specific cell-receptor susceptibility in female patients with uncomplicated recurrent urinary tract infections. Type I, or mannose-sensitive, fimbriae are important in initiating colonization of the bladder. Certainly *E. coli* possessing type I fimbriae are found more often in patients with UTI. Blood group antigens, carbohydrate structures bound to lipids or proteins, make up the key component of the uroepithelial cell membrane where bacteria affix. A blood group antigen expression on vaginal cells and mucus in women with recurrent infections may be a factor, but Navas et al. (9) found no significant differences in ABH or Lewis antigen blood group expression between patient and control groups, even when controlling for ABO or secretor phenotypes. Women who have frequently recurrent disease were thought to be non-secretors of the ABO blood type groups.

Fimbriated cell-wall extensions (pili) allow bacteria to attach to the glycoprotein receptors of urothelial cells. Patients with repeated episodes of pyelonephritis and renal failure have been found to have higher P-fimbriae receptor accessiblity on uroepithelial cells than individuals with repeated pyelonephritis and normal renal function. Properties of bacterial endotoxin secretion assist the microorganism to attach and invade. Endotoxin causes inhibition of ureteral motility and could explain some features of intrarenal reflux and invasion at the level of the renal papillae. *E. coli* accounts for more than 80% of acute uncomplicated pyelonephritis in young women. Uropathogenic bacteria belong to a small number of O:K:H serotypic groups and produce hemolysin and aerobactin as well as possess the pyelonephritis-associated pili. About 30% of these organisms are resistant to amoxicillin and first-generation cephalosporins.

DIAGNOSIS AND TREATMENT IN THE MANAGED CARE ERA

It is obvious that a tremendous amount of socioeconomic pressure is being generated to streamline and reduce the cost of health care delivery. Given the prevalence of urinary tract infections, every effort to simplify the treatment and reduce the morbidity and its consequent costs of lost work as well as further expenditure of health care dollars on complications must be made.

Specimen Collection

The difficulty with most diagnostic evaluation for urinary tract infections lies with the method of collecting the specimen. That duty is usually left to the least-trained individual, often the patient, in the office or clinic area. Most times the specimen is sent off to a laboratory technician, and the physician has no supervisory or evaluation role whatsoever. The cost of unnecessary urine cultures and full-spectrum urinalysis can be avoided by having the physician taking fewer than 60 seconds to do a dipstick test and microscopy of a spun urine sediment. The physician should be quite certain of the technique for urine collection and should instruct the patient in careful collecting technique. In obese women, some infants, and many individuals with neurogenic bladder, a suprapubic aspiration is by far the best method for accuracy in colony counts, organism qualification, and evaluation of leukocytes.

The initial diagnostic testing and clinical evaluation of the patient sets the pattern for management of the urinary tract infection. The individual treatment approach may mean the difference between resolving a symptomatic infection or dealing with recurrence or persistent infection. Even how the physician instructs the patient in taking the medication may determine the course of outcome; patients notoriously fail to complete a full course of antibiotic therapy, stopping when they feel better. A level of suspicion for complicating factors in that particular host needs to be kept in mind. As we evolve in our managed care milieu and have computerized models of outcomes analysis superimposed on our practice, we will have to define patient characteristics more accurately, quantify and identify organisms and leukocyte and systemic response to infection in the urine and blood stream, and adhere to carefully systematized clinical treatment pathways. This is undoubtedly better for the patient and the health care expenditure dollar. These kinds of careful evaluation of patients and their infections have already been worked on in consensus conference as a systematic catalog (10). Utilizing such careful scrutiny and descriptive criteria will enhance any clinical studies regarding treatment and new drug trials.

Uroradiological Investigation

When a UTI has been characterized and fitted into one of the categories mentioned above, the natural evolution of evaluation may recommend radiologic or urologic interventional testing. Clearly, to detect the presence of vesicoureteral reflux in the child with UTI is valuable. Routine uroradiologic evaluation in uncomplicated young women is unwarranted. By simply assessing the category of infection, the reflex usage of ancillary testing and consequent costs can be avoided.

Laboratory Evaluation of UTI

Despite the existence of many available systems for the detection of pyuria and bacteriuria, the accurate diagnosis of urinary tract infection remains problematic. There are varying sensitivities for detecting colony-forming bacteria, and they do well with $>10^4$ organism count but begin to fall short with lesser numbers of bacteria. The same is true for the enzymatic leukocyte-detecting dipsticks. In a recent study of urinary screening methods, the Chemstrip 9 revealed a 67% sensitivity with 98% specificity for leukocyte esterase and nitrate (11). The Uriscreen showed 92% sensitivity and 89% specificity. Methylene blue stain and Gram stain for pyuria were not as sensitive for either pyuria or bacteriuria as these chemical tests.

Most workers agree that a urinary tract infection, as opposed to colonization, is represented by a host response in the form of leukocyte excretion. Typically, a urinary tract infection causes an immune response and neutrophil excretion on the order of 400,000 cells per hour and estimated as >10 WBCs/HPF of a spun sediment. A 10-ml sample of urine centrifuged at 2,000 rpm for a minimum of 2 to 5 minutes has been the typical analysis in a busy office. More accuracy would be gained by using a hemacytometer to count unspun urine leukocytes as >10 WBCs/mm^3. Unspun urine in a counting chamber has a high sensitivity and less variability in results. A counting chamber such as the KOVA slide is inexpensive and disposable. The coefficient of variation (CV) reveals that a resuspended sediment analysis for pyuria varies 43%, while a counting chamber is in the 10–25% variable range; 90–95% of patients with >10 WBCs/mm^3 are proved to have significant bacteriuria.

The bioluminescence assay that detects bacterial ATP appears to have true clinical value in detecting significant bacteriuria. Set against the reference of routinely cultured urine specimens, the bioluminescence screening scored a 93% sensitivity, a 78% specificity, and a 99% predictive accuracy for negative results. When compared with the routine dipsticks for nitrites and leukocyte esterase, the sensitivities of 54% and 59%, respectively, were a poor second place (12).

Significant Bacteriuria

Urinary tract infection usually implies the presence of symptoms, but in some cases one can have bacteria colonizing the urinary tract and be asymptomatic. In other cases there can be invasion of the urinary tract tissues with pyuria and immune response and still no significant symptoms. Patients with sensory deprivation and neurogenic bladder are representative of this group. In specific instances this condition warrants therapy.

The concept of significant bacteriuria was established many years ago and was based on the ability of *E. coli*, for example, to grow rapidly in urine. The organism could achieve high densities within 8 to 12 hours. For this reason, using $>10^5$ organisms as a validated infection count was adopted as useful and consistent. Counts of 10^2 to 10^4 CFU/ml are significant when combined with symptoms and pyuria. No difference in outcome of treatment occurs between the two groups. Many with low counts are treated empirically with antimicrobials. The standard for infection should be $>10^3$ if an approriate midstream urine is obtained—that is, by a nurse. A catheterized or suprapubic specimen is also adequate to define such a level of bacteriuria.

Recurrent Infection

It is extremely difficult for us to be precise in identifying recurrence/persistence or, as in 90% of the cases, reinfection as the problem in the patient with unresolved urinary tract infection. Without doing serotyping or DNA studies, it becomes a microbiologic nightmare. This kind of sophistication in laboratory analysis is also expensive. Low-count bacteriuria may be an early phase of infection, possibly localized to the urethra. We are also becoming aware that *Staphylococcus saprophyticus* is an important organism in young women and may be responsible for low counts and low WBCs in the urine.

Selection of Antimicrobial Treatment

Most therapeutic intervention occurs because the patient presents with signs and symptoms of urinary tract infection. We rely on the presence of pyuria and documentation of significant amounts of pathogenic bacteria on culture to confirm our impression of significant infection. This is not to say that patients cannot have symptoms, and even pyuria, in the absence of virulent microorganisms. It behooves the physician, however, to investigate further if bacteria cannot be demonstrated. Therapy is less often indicated for the treatment of asymptomatic bacteriuria.

Antimicrobial treatment regimens should be considered for curative effect, prophylaxis, or suppression. Most of the past treatment regimens have advocated too much antibiotic for too long a time.

A rationale for treatment is important. If one adheres to the categories of infection set out, uncomplicated infection in premenopausal women over the age of 16 should receive the simplest treatment. It has been shown repeatedly that 85–100% of these infections respond to a single-dose regimen, but some mitigating circumstances have pushed the community of physicians studying UTI to suggest that a 3-day regimen should be the empiric choice for this category. Trimethoprim or trimethoprim/sulfamethoxazole is a good choice in these individuals who are unlikely to have resistant organisms. Adverse reactions are few with such a short course, and 95% of women are predictably cured. Trimethoprim alone can be used in those sensitive to sulfonamide. Amoxicillin or ampicillin is no longer a good choice for first-line treatment because of the high incidence (30%) of natural resistance in the community. Oral cephalosporins such as cephalexin are also good choices and safe in pregnancy.

For the treatment of women with acute uncomplicated pyelonephritis, it is valuable to give a single-dose loading therapy to wash out bacteria; 200 mg gentamicin, for example, followed by appropriate oral medication. The duration of antimicrobial treatment in uncomplicated acute pyelonephritis has been too long and in some cases with combination therapy in the past. Five days is adequate for excellent outcomes in uncomplicated pyelonephritis of young women. After intravenous initiation and hydration, oral outpatient therapy is adequate. Oral medications would be used only if the patients have no nausea and vomiting; otherwise they may need intravenous therapy for a 48- to 72-hour period. There is no evidence that combinations of antibiotics are more effective in treating these uncomplicated pyelonephritis episodes. Combination ampicillin should probably be dropped from the initial loading dose of treatment. Other appropriate parenteral antimicrobial choices for initial treatment of uncomplicated pyelonephritis include the β-lactams and fluoroquinolones. Single daily dosing is now available for all of these agents.

Clinical vs. Microbiological Efficacy

Clinical cure implies that symptoms and pyuria disappear; microbiologic cure is more problematic. We probably should not accept any residual count, no matter how low, as a cure.

How Should Treatment Vary for the Pediatric Population?

Age is one of the most important factors in determining treatment in the pediatric population. Patients should be categorized as neonates, infants, or children. Neonates are up to 6 months old, and infants are under 1 year of age. Because symptoms are difficult to assess, one relies on fever and white cell count. Acute uncomplicated pyelonephritis inevitably has fever as a sign.

Methods of urine collection are problematic. In neonates, infants, and young children, suprapubic aspiration is the only acceptable method for collecting samples. Sometimes one can do some stroking or otherwise induce a small breast- or bottle-feeding infant to void and then catch a midstream specimen.

Dosing

Single-dose therapy has not been used extensively and is poorly investigated in the pediatric age group. There are obvious benefits of single-dose therapy in this group. Single-dose therapy causes significantly less suppression of the rectal and periurethral flora. Compliance obviously is less of an issue. One study utilizing a single dose of gentamicin vs. an oral 7-day conventional course showed no difference in outcome provided one was dealing with an uncomplicated, nonrecurrent infection (13). Most physicians subscribe to the current standard of care for uncomplicated infections at the present time as 3 days, and prophylaxis may be indicated for those suffering two or more infections in a 6-month period. Treatment time for pyelonephritis in children should be 3 to 5 days of intravenous antimicrobial therapy; they should then be switched to oral treatment. There are no data to support the 10 days of intravenous therapy often administered by pediatricians.

There is general agreement that infants and children who develop urinary tract infection—usually pyelonephritis—should undergo urinary tract investigation because a high proportion of them have abnormalities.

In some refractory recurrent infection problems, success has been achieved utilizing double antimicrobial prophylaxis (14) nitrofurantoin 2 mg/kg each morning and trimethoprim with or without sulfamethoxazole 2/10 mg/kg at bedtime. The children in this report were suffering from reflux (68%) and detrusor instability/voiding dysfunction (49%).

Children do suffer from significant urinary tract infections caused by gram-positive organisms, and there are reports of pyelonephritis caused by *Staphylococcus epidermidis* (15).

RECURRENT UTI AND PROPHYLAXIS IN THE UNCOMPLICATED HOST

Once the commitment to prophylaxis of recurrent infection in either the uncomplicated or complicated patient has been made, the choice of

TABLE 1. *Summary of suggested prophylaxis protocols for various forms of complicated urinary tract infection*

Patients/ Infection	Recommended antimicrobials	Daily dosing	Duration
Premenopausal woman, uncomplicated recurrent	nitrofurantoin trimethoprim/sulfa cephalexin	50 mg hs 40/80 mg hs 125 mg hs or after coitus	6 months
Pediatric population	nitrofurantoin trimethoprim/sulfa	2 mg/kg hs 2 mg/kg hs	6 months
Pregnant women (asymptomatic & pyelo)	nitrofurantoin	50 mg hs	Ad lib until term
Symptomatic diabetes and elderly (recurrent pyelo)	nitrofurantoin	100 mg hs	Indefinite
	trimethoprim/sulfa cephalexin fluoroquinolone vaginal estrogen cream	80/160 mg hs 250 mg hs 400 mg hs nightly	
Neurogenic bladder	nitrofurantoin trimethoprim/sulfa cephalexin intravesical neomycin/ polymixin	100 mg qd 80/160 mg qd 250 mg qd 4 vials per liter saline 30 cc per cath	Indefinite
Proteus struvite calculus	penicillin G	500 mg bid	Suppression
Chronic bacterial prostatitis (therapeutic)	fluoroquinolone	400 mg bid	3 months

antimicrobial agent and dosing is optional (Table 1). In the sexually active young woman, postcoital antimicrobial management works very well. In some individuals the decision will be to use a nightly dose of medication, and in the very sophisticated patient, self-start treatment may be preferred to prophylaxis.

Postmenopausal women may benefit from topical estrogen. A recent double-blinded controlled study of 93 postmenopausal women showed a good outcome when followed for 8 months (16). The incidence of recurrent urinary infection in the group with estrogen was significantly reduced. There were 0.5 vs. 5.9 episodes per patient-year. Lactobacilli were absent in all vaginal cultures before treatment and reappeared after one month in 22 of 36 estriol-treated women but in none of the 24 placebo recipients. With estriol, the mean vaginal pH declined from 5.5 to 3.8 (p <0.001).

Bacterial extract oral immunotherapy is another non-antimicrobial approach to recurrent infection (17). Patients were treated with an immunostimulating bacterial extract once daily for 3 months. This therapy was significantly superior to placebo in reducing recurrent infection.

UTI OF PREGNANCY

There is no question that when a pregnant woman is found to have asymptomatic bacteriuria, she has a higher likelihood of suffering from acute pyelonephritis of pregnancy. Approximately 5% of pregnant women have asymptomatic bacteriuria, and 15–40% of these develop acute pyelonephritis, usually during the last trimester. Clinical trials have demonstrated the usefulness of an initial trial of single- or short-course therapy in these individuals as long as the follow-up culture shows absence of bacteria. These women need to have repeated cultures at each clinical visit. If they relapse and fail a second short course of therapy, they should then be put on prophylaxis, such as nitrofurantoin 50 mg nightly. Pregnant women with acute uncomplicated pyelonephritis should be treated the same way as women who are not pregnant. Women who have a history of developing recurrent urinary tract infections have been equally successful in avoiding infections during pregnancy using postcoital or nightly prophylaxis (18). It is desirable to give a pregnant woman the lowest effective dose of a drug and for a very short time period. It is probably adequate to consider even single-dose therapy (19,20).

UTI AND DIABETES MELLITUS

Diabetic patients represent a large proportion of those individuals labeled as suffering from complicated UTI. It is estimated that the occurrence of infection in women with diabetes is two to three times greater than in a similar age group of women without the metabolic disorder. The same is not true for men, where the prevalence of bacteriuria is the same regardless of the presence of diabetes. But just as most men suffer upper-tract infection, so do the majority of women with diabetes who develop bacterial invasion. It is estimated that the incidence of acute pyelonephritis may be as much as five times that of nondiabetic patients; similarly there is more likelihood of bilateral pyelonephritis.

Any physician caring for a diabetic patient with UTI must constantly be vigilant and not miss intrarenal abscess, urinary tract emphysema, perinephric abscess, papillary necrosis, and other invasive tissue infections. Many times these have less than an impressive clinical presentation for their size and complexity; nevertheless, the morbidity and mortality rates continue to be high. Even when the patient does not appear to be systemically ill, high peripheral white cell counts and significant pyuria will be seen. Blood cultures should always be obtained. Early institution of intravenous antimicrobial therapy and hydration may help avoid some of the progressive invasive complications. The primary care physician must always maintain a high level of concern for these individuals when a UTI is suspected.

Bladder dysfunction with poor emptying appears to be the most likely underlying basis for an increased colonization rate in diabetics. Some studies have also suggested that glycosuria inhibits efficient leukocyte function. Because of the higher incidence of asymptomatic bacteriuria and devastating invasion when out of control, many have suggested that these cases of asymptomatic bacteriuria be treated, much as we suggest that pregnant women have their asymptomatic colonization eradicated.

Treatment of symptomatic infections in the diabetic patient cannot be limited to a 3-day course as in uncomplicated cystitis; rather, the 7- to 14-day course of treatment will help eradicate the upper-tract colonization. There does not appear to be any benefit from prolonged (6-week) therapy. *E. coli* is the most common organism involved in diabetic UTI, but *Klebsiella* and *Proteus* are also commonly found. Fungal infections are also found and are discussed in Chapter 8. Trimethoprim/sulfamethoxazole is a good first-line therapy for those patients having cystitis. In more complex settings the fluoroquinolones have an excellent track record. The enterococcus organisms need to be treated with one of the penicillins.

REFERENCES

1. Schappert SM. National ambulatory medical care survey: 1991. Hyattsville, Maryland: National Center for Health Statistics; 1992.
2. Platt R, Polk BF, Murdock B, Rosner B. Mortality associated with nosocomial urinary tract infection. *New Engl J Med* 1992;307:637.
3. Kawada Y. Inclusion criteria for acute uncomplicated cystitis. *Infection* 1992;20(Suppl 3):S143.
4. Schaeffer AJ. Diagnostics and categories of patients. *Infection* 1992;20(Suppl 3):S138.
5. Bryan CS, Reynolds KL. Hospital-acquired bacteremic urinary tract infection: epidemiology and outcome. *J Urol* 1982;132:494.
6. Jerkeman M, Braconier JH. Bacteremic and non-bacteremic febrile urinary tract infection—a review of 168 hospital-treated patients. *Infection* 1992;20:143.
7. Kawada Y. Comparison of complicated urinary tract infections in men and women. *Infection* 1992;22(Suppl 1):S55.
8. Schaeffer AJ, Jones JM, Dunn JK. Association of in vitro Escherichia coli adherence to vaginal and buccal epithelial cells with susceptibility of women to recurrent urinary tract infections. *New Engl J Med* 1981;304:1062.
9. Navas EI, Venegas MF, Duncan JL, Anderson BE, Kanerva C, Chmiel JS, Schaeffer AJ. Blood group antigen expression on vaginal cells and mucus in women with and without a history of urinary tract infections. *J Urol* 1994;152:345.
10. Naber KG. Characteristics of patients with urinary tract infections. *Infection* 1992;20(Suppl 3):S145.
11. Carroll KC, Hale DC, Von Boerum DH, Reich GC, Hamilton LT, Matsen JM. Laboratory evaluation of urinary tract infections in an ambulatory clinic. *Am J Clin Path* 1994;101:100.
12. Graninger W, Fleischmann D, Schneeweiss B, Aram L, Stockenhumber F. Rapid screening for bacteriuria in pregnancy. *Infection* 1992;20:9–11.

13. Grimwood K, Abbott GD, Fergusson DM. Single dose gentamicin in treatment of urinary tract infections in children. *NZ Med J* 1988;101:539.
14. Smith EM, Elder JS. Double antimicrobial prophylaxis in girls with breakthrough urinary tract infections. *Urology* 1994;43:708.
15. Hall DE, Snitzer JA. Staphylococcus epidermidis as a cause of urinary tract infection in children. *J Pediatr* 1994;124:437.
16. Rax R, Stamm WE. A controlled trial of intravaginal estriol in postmenopausal women with recurrent urinary tract infections. *New Engl J Med* 1993;329:753.
17. Schulman CC, Corbusier A, Michiels H, Taenzer HJ. Oral immunotherapy of recurrent urinary tract infections: a double-blind, placebo-controlled multicenter study. *J Urol* 1993;150:917.
18. Pfau A, Sacks TG. Effective prophylaxis for recurrent urinary tract infection during pregnancy. *Clin Infect Dis* 1992;14:810.
19. Bailey RR, Bishop V, Peddie BA. Comparison of single dose with a 5-day course of co-trimoxazole for asymptomatic (covert) bacteriuria of pregnancy. *Aust N Z J Obstet Gynaecol* 1983;23:139.
20. Tan JS, File TM Jr. Treatment of bacteriuria in pregnancy. *Drugs* 1992;44:972.

Antibiotic Therapy in Urology,
edited by S. Grant Mulholland, M.D.,
Lippincott-Raven Publishers, Philadelphia © 1996.

Chapter 4

Bacteriuria and Urinary Tract Infections in the Elderly

Lindsay E. Nicolle

Departments of Medicine and Medical Microbiology, University of Manitoba, MS-675 Health Sciences Centre, Manitoba R3A 1R9 Canada

The populations of developed countries continue to age. Medical problems associated with aging will become increasingly important over the next several decades. Urinary tract infection is the most frequent bacterial infection in the elderly. A thorough understanding of urinary infection in the elderly and its optimal management will be essential to provide care to our increasingly older populations.

The elderly population is not homogeneous. A spectrum of health status varies from the well, ambulant individual who has no physical impairment and is socially and financially secure to the fully dependent, noncommunicative, long-term care resident maintained with feeding tubes, indwelling Foley catheters, and long-term respirator therapy. The clinical relevance and management of urinary infection vary with the spectrum of functional impairment and comorbidities of different elderly populations.

In the United States, it has been reported that as many as 43% of all individuals who reached age 65 in 1990 will reside in a long-term care institution at some time before their death (1). This institutionalized population has an extraordinary prevalence and incidence of urinary infection (2). Institutionalization amplifies transmission of organisms among individuals, and, because of intense antimicrobial use, promotes emergence of antimicrobial resistance. Thus, appropriate management of urinary infection, including optimal approaches to antimicrobial use, is of particular importance for these populations. Generally, 5–10% of the institutionalized elderly have long-term indwelling catheters. Such patients are unique in many aspects with respect to urinary infection. Several recent reviews have discussed long-term catheter use in the elderly in detail (3,4). This chapter discusses aspects relevant only to noncatheterized elderly populations, unless otherwise stated.

TABLE 1. *Prevalence of asymptomatic bacteriuria in different institutionalized populations without long-term indwelling catheters*

	Prevalence	
Population (reference)	Women	Men
United States: >70 y, Veteran's hospital (11)		31%
United States: extended care (12)	17%	26%
United States: nursing home (10)	23%	
Canada: long-term care (14,15)	55%	37%
Denmark: long-term care (16)	42%	15%
Scotland: geriatric assessment (17)	34%	31%
Greece: home for elderly (13)	27%	19%

OCCURRENCE

Increasing prevalence of bacteriuria with increasing age has been consistently reported for both men and women in different populations. For women over 60, community studies report a prevalence of bacteriuria of 5–10%, increasing to as much as 20–30% in the oldest age groups (5–11). This compares with a prevalence of less than 5% in young women. For men, the prevalence of bacteriuria in the community population is lower than that reported for women, but generally 5–10% of those over 70 years are reported to have bacteriuria (5,9,11,12). Institutionalized populations have a remarkable prevalence of bacteriuria (Table 1). From 17–55% of women and 15–31% of men are bacteriuric (2). Among the most highly functionally disabled in these institutions, the prevalence of bacteriuria is over 50% for both men and women.

There is also a high incidence of bacteriuria in the elderly. Boscia et al. (5) reported that 18% of women and 6% of men in an elderly ambulatory American population had bacteriuria at initial screening. The cumulative prevalence at 18 months, with screening every 6 months, was 10% for men and 30% for women. Kasviki-Charvati et al. (13) reported rates of "turnover" of bacteriuria in ambulant men and women in an elderly residential home in Athens. Eleven percent of men and 23% of women with negative urine cultures at admission to the facility had at least one positive urine culture by 12 months. They also reported that 22% of men and 27% of women bacteriuric at admission were not bacteriuric at 12 months. Abrutyn et al. (10) reported similar observations in elderly women, with the incidence of bacteriuria in institutionalized women higher than that in an ambulant geriatric apartment population. In a group of highly functionally impaired elderly institutionalized men, the incidence of new infections was 45/100 patient-years, with 10% of previously nonbacteriuric subjects acquiring bacteriuria in any 3-month period (14). For a similarly impaired population of institutionalized elderly women, the incidence of infections was 1.2 per resident-year (15).

MICROBIOLOGY

Representative reports of the microbiology of bacteriuria in the elderly are summarized in Table 2. This information is obtained from prevalence studies in asymptomatic elderly populations; the microbiology of symptomatic infection is not as well studied. For the noninstitutionalized elderly, *Escherichia coli* is the single most frequent organism isolated, but there appears to be an increased prevalence of gram-positive organisms, such as coagulase-negative staphylococci, *Streptococcus faecalis*, and group B streptococci (5). *Proteus mirabilis* and *Klebsiella pneumoniae* are the most frequent gram-negative organisms isolated after *Escherichia coli*. In institutionalized women, *E. coli* remains the most frequent organism. For men, however, *P. mirabilis* occurs with greatest frequency, with *E. coli* second (2). Gram-negative organisms that may have increased antimicrobial resistance are isolated more frequently in institutionalized populations (18). These include *Pseudomonas aeruginosa*, *Providencia stuartii*, *Citrobacter freundii*, and *Enterobacter cloacae*. This likely reflects the intensive antimicrobial exposure in long-term care facilities, including repeated antimicrobial courses in individual patients. Mixed infections occur frequently in the institutionalized population and are reported in 10–25% of bacteriuric subjects (2).

TABLE 2. *Representative reports of infecting organisms isolated from elderly subjects with asymptomatic bacteriuria*

	Ambulant		Institutionalized	
	Women (5)[a]	Men (5)	Women (15)	Men (14)
Escherichia coli	54	3	30	13
Proteus mirabilis	1		14	36
Pseudomonas aeruginosa				23
Klebsiella pneumoniae	8			7
Providencia spp				19
Morganella morganii				3
Enterobacter aerogenes		1	11	2
Citrobacter spp				3
Other gram-negative				
Enterococcus spp	1	4		6
Group B streptococci	3			2
Staphylococcus aureus			2	3
Coagulase-negative staphylococci		1		2
Other gram-positive				

[a]Numbers in parentheses refer to references.

Urinary infection is the most frequent source of bacteremia in the elderly (19–23), with over 50% of episodes consistently reported to be of a urinary source. *E. coli* is the principal organism isolated from bacteremic infection in most series. The distribution of organisms in bacteremic urinary infection may differ from the bacteriology of urinary infection, suggesting certain organisms, particularly *E. coli*, may have unique virulence (22). Many reviews of bacteremia in nursing homes do not differentiate between bacteremic patients with and without long-term indwelling catheters.

Potential difficulties in urine specimen collection in elderly populations must be addressed. For the well, ambulant, noninstitutionalized elderly, adequate voided specimens can usually be obtained from both men and women. For the diagnosis of asymptomatic bacteriuria in men, one voided specimen is generally sufficient (24). Two consecutive specimens with the same organism in quantitative counts of $>10^5$ colony forming units (CFU)/ml are required to diagnose asymptomatic bacteriuria in women. For symptomatic infection, one specimen is sufficient. Functional impairment and comorbid illnesses in the institutionalized population result in a failure to obtain adequate voided specimens from some subjects. Valid specimens can be collected through external condom collecting devices in men if a standardized collection procedure is followed to minimize contamination (25,26). Highly impaired institutionalized women may not be able to provide voided specimens (15). Where there is a clear indication for obtaining a urine specimen and it is unlikely a voided specimen can be collected without contamination, the specimen should be obtained through in-and-out catheterization. Straight catheterization itself, however, is associated with acquisition of bacteriuria in as many as 5% of episodes.

PATHOGENESIS OF URINARY INFECTION

The usual means of infection acquisition is the ascending route from the periurethral area to the bladder and, in some cases, subsequently the kidney. The gastrointestinal tract is a reservoir for potentially infecting organisms. For women, there is a change in the vaginal and periurethral flora in the postmenopausal period caused by the loss of endogenous estrogen (27). This leads to increased vaginal and periurethral colonization with *E. coli* and other Enterobacteriaceae, perhaps contributing to the increased frequency of urinary infection in postmenopausal women. The most important factor promoting bacteriuria in men is prostatic hypertrophy, which leads to urethral obstruction, impaired voiding, and increased post-void residual (PVR) urine volumes. The bactericidal activity of prostatic fluid is decreased in older men (28), but whether this contributes to bacteriuria is unknown. Men with incontinence managed by external drainage devices (condom catheter and leg bag) are at increased risk for urinary infection (29). These devices frequently have heavy periuretheral colonization with gram-negative organisms. With obstruction of urinary drainage because of kinking or twisting of the condom or drainage tube, urinary infection may occur (29).

Comorbid illness is likely the major factor promoting acquisition of bacteriuria in the institutionalized elderly (2). Many neurologic illnesses that occur with increased frequency in the elderly and may in themselves lead to a requirement for institutional care are associated with a neurogenic bladder. These include Alzheimer's disease, Parkinson's disease, and cerebrovascular accidents. The neurogenic bladder is associated with impaired voiding, increased residual volume, and an increased frequency of ureteric reflux.

Over 50% of asymptomatic infections in elderly institutionalized women are localized to the kidney (30,31). Women of older age and longer institutionalization are more likely to have renal localization (31). Kidney infection is less likely to be eradicated with usual antimicrobial regimens than bladder infection. A high proportion of men have prostatic infection (14). The prostate provides a protected environment into which most antimicrobials penetrate poorly. Infected prostatic stones are an additional niche from which bacteria cannot be eradicated. Bacterial infection of the prostate frequently leads to relapsing urinary infection. Any duration of antimicrobial therapy may be ineffective in eradicating bacteria from this focus. An increased frequency of relapsing renal and prostatic infection in older populations also increases the overall prevalence of bacteriuria.

HOST-ORGANISM INTERACTIONS

Most bacteriuric elderly are asymptomatic. Symptomatic infections, when they occur, appear to have characteristics of organism virulence factors and host response similar to those of younger populations. Organisms isolated from cases of symptomatic infection have a higher frequency of virulence factors than those isolated from cases of asymptomatic bacteriuria (32,33). For instance, *E. coli* are more likely to express the P-pilus and be hemolytic, and less likely to be rough strains relatively deficient in lipopolysaccharide. Obstruction of urine drainage or trauma to the bacteriuric urinary tract, however, leads to invasive infection independent of organism virulence factors.

Most elderly subjects with asymptomatic urinary infection have evidence for a host response as measured by pyuria (26,31,34,35). Over 90% of elderly men or women with asymptomatic bacteriuria have associated pyuria (26,31). In addition, as many as 30% of elderly institutionalized subjects without bacteriuria also have pyuria (34,35). The almost universal occurrence of pyuria among the asymptomatic bacteriuric elderly suggests that attempts to differentiate "colonization" from "infection" on the basis of the presence or absence of pyuria are not valid.

In addition to pyuria, elderly subjects with asymptomatic bacteriuria show a spectrum of local urinary immune and inflammatory responses. From one-third to one-half of institutionalized bacteriuric elderly subjects have an elevated level of urinary antibody to uropathogens as compared with nonbacteriuric subjects (36). In addition, from 25–50% have measurable urinary interleukin-6 or urinary interleukin-1α (37). Both of these cytokines occur significantly more frequently in subjects with asymptomatic bacteriuria as compared with subjects without bacteriuria. Some elderly individuals with asymptomatic bacteriuria also have evidence for an ongoing systemic response, as manifested by an increased level of serum antibody to the potential uropathogens (36,38). Factors that influence the degree of host response are not yet described.

Elderly individuals with invasive infection have a systemic response to the infection (38). This includes increased level of antibody to the infecting uropathogen, elevated C-reactive protein, and elevated serum interleukin-6 levels (unpublished observations). Limited published reports to date do not suggest consistent qualitative or quantitative differences in response in the elderly as compared with a younger population with invasive urinary infection.

CLINICAL IMPACT

Morbidity of Urinary Infection

Symptomatic urinary infection in the elderly may present with clinical symptoms similar to those in younger populations (Table 3). These may be primarily irritative symptoms, such as dysuria, urgency, and frequency, as well as alterations in continence status. Pyelonephritis may present with classic manifestations of fever and costovertebral angle pain and tenderness. Other presentations in this population include epididymo-orchitis, urethritis, or urethral abscesses in men. These occur more frequently in subjects maintained on long-term indwelling catheters or in men with external urinary drainage devices.

There are few population-based studies that define the morbidity of urinary infection in the noninstitutionalized elderly. Irvine et al. (39) found that 3% of hospitalizations from a geriatric outpatient clinic were for genitourinary infection, and Gleckman et al. (20) reported that uri-

TABLE 3. *Symptomatic manifestations possibly attributable to urinary infection in elderly subjects*

Probable/possible	Unlikely
Acute irritative symptoms: dysuria, frequency, urgency, increased incontinence	Chronic genitourinary symptoms
Fever with localizing genitourinary symptoms	Fever without localizing genitourinary symptoms
Acute pyelonephritis	Nonspecific decline
Epididymo-orchitis	Gross hematuria
Urethral abscess	
Urethritis (with catheter)	

nary infection is the most common cause of gram-negative bacteremia in elderly patients admitted to a hospital. Gram-negative bacteremia resulting from urinary infection was, however, responsible for fewer than 1% of all admissions of elderly subjects. Boscia et al. (40) reported that 16% of 61 women with asymptomatic bacteriuria in a geriatric apartment setting became symptomatic in follow-up, but did not specify the severity of symptomatic episodes. There is no evidence to suggest that urinary infection contributes to renal failure in this population.

The high prevalence of chronic genitourinary symptoms in the institutionalized population complicates the assessment of morbidity from urinary infection. These chronic genitourinary symptoms include incontinence, frequency, dysuria, and urgency. Chronic genitourinary symptoms and nonspecific general complaints without localizing genitourinary symptoms are not the consequence of urinary infection, although many of these individuals are bacteriuric (41,42). Boscia et al. (42) demonstrated that women had a similar frequency of such symptoms when their urine cultures were bacteriuric or sterile. Berman et al. (43) reported that 9.2% of episodes of "general decline" in an institutionalized population were caused by urinary infection. All subjects with urinary infection were febrile. It was not stated how many of these patients had long-term indwelling catheters.

Attempts to define the morbidity attributable to urinary infection in the institutionalized elderly are compromised by the high prevalence of bacteriuria in this population. Where the prevalence of bacteriuria is 20–50%, any patient with a fever has a high likelihood of a positive urine culture (2). In this situation a fever with a positive urine culture has low predictive value for a diagnosis of invasive urinary infection.

The contribution of urinary infection to morbidity in the institutionalized elderly is small relative to the high prevalence and incidence of bacteriuria (44). In prospective studies of infectious morbidity in elderly populations, symptomatic urinary tract infection occurs relatively infrequently, although the incidence is increased in individuals with long-term indwelling catheters. Respiratory tract infections, including pneumonia, fevers of unknown source, and skin and soft tissue infections occur more frequently than symptomatic urinary infection (44,45).

Several studies have used clinical criteria in an attempt to estimate morbidity associated with bacteriuria. In institutionalized subjects, rates of symptomatic infection of 0.11–0.15 per bacteriuric year have been reported (14,15). Urinary infection is reported as the reason for transfer from nursing homes to acute care facilities in 1–8% of episodes (39,46). Again, the contribution of long-term indwelling catheters was not stated. In a prospective study using clinical or serologic criteria for identification of invasive urinary infection in the institutionalized elderly, fewer than 10% of episodes of fever were caused by urinary tract infection (47).

Urinary infection is the most common cause of bacteremia for both noninstitutionalized and institutionalized elderly populations (19–23). Elderly women with pyelonephritis are more frequently bacteremic than younger women (20). Bacteremic urinary infection may further be complicated by metastatic infection at other sites, including prosthetic devices, or endocarditis (48).

Gross hematuria is frequently ascribed to hemorrhagic cystitis in the elderly and treated as urinary infection. It is more frequently identified in men (49). A prospective descriptive study of gross hematuria in residents of long-term care facilities identified bacteriuria in 75% of episodes (49). Clinical evidence, however, was not consistent with hemorrhagic cystitis caused by urinary infection contributing to these episodes. Most individuals had other diagnoses to explain gross hematuria, including indwelling catheters, diverticuli, stones, and tumors.

Other potential "morbidity" in the incontinent institutionalized population includes unpleasant urinary odor and the contribution of bacteriuria to decubitus ulcer infection. Urinary infection may be associated with an offensive odor, likely caused by bacterial polyamine production, but this is not universal. We found that 78% of urines judged by the nursing staff in one long-term care facility to be offensively malodorous were bacteriuric, but 35% of nonmalodorous urines were also bacteriuric (50). In a 2-year prospective study of decubitus ulcers in residents of two large nursing homes, no episodes of infected decubitus ulcers with the same organism isolated from the urinary tract and the infected pressure sore were identified, although decubitus infection occurred infrequently (51). The urinary isolate was identified as a colonizing organism of the decubitus ulcer in fewer than 5% of noninfected ulcers, with specimens obtained monthly. Thus, under usual standards of nursing home care, urinary infection does not contribute to morbidity of infected decubitus ulcers.

Mortality

Initial reports from Greece (52) and Finland (53) suggested asymptomatic bacteriuria in the ambulant elderly was associated with decreased survival in both men and women. In these studies, however, no explanation for this association was apparent. Subsequent studies performed in community populations in both Sweden (9) and Finland (54) failed to confirm this association. In the Swedish study, elderly men with bacteriuria had poorer survival, but this observation did not persist when corrected for the presence of genitourinary malignancy (9). Prospective studies in institutionalized populations have failed to find evidence for increased mortality in bacteriuric residents (55,56). Currently, there is no compelling evidence supporting a causal relationship between asymptomatic bacteriuria and mortality in the elderly.

Acute invasive urinary infection, with or without bacteremia, may lead to septic shock and death. Despite urinary infection being the most frequent cause of bacteremia in elderly populations, urinary infection is infrequently a direct cause of death. The case fatality ratio is less than 10% for bacteremia of a urinary source (19,21). Autopsy series of elderly subjects report urinary infection as a cause of death in fewer than 1% of cases (55,57,58). In fact, these studies show that the only infection associated with substantial mortality in the elderly is pneumonia.

THERAPY OF URINARY INFECTION IN THE ELDERLY

Urinary infection is the most frequent reason for antimicrobial administration in residents of long-term care facilities (59–61). Given the relatively limited morbidity identified with urinary infection, it would seem that much of this antimicrobial use may not be appropriate. Studies have, in fact, reported that over 50% of antimicrobial use for urinary infection in the institutionalized elderly is inappropriate (60,61). Characteristics of antimicrobial use for urinary infection have not been described for elderly individuals in the community.

Asymptomatic Bacteriuria

Several prospective randomized studies have compared treatment to nontreatment for asymptomatic bacteriuria in elderly populations (14,15,40,56).

In the study of Boscia et al. (40), elderly women resident in a geriatric apartment were randomized to receive treatment with a 3-day course of trimethoprim or no therapy. The treated group had a significant decrease in the prevalence of asymptomatic bacteriuria at 6 months, from 60% with no therapy to 30% in treated subjects. There was also a decrease in symptomatic episodes in the 6-month period subsequent to therapy, with 16 episodes identified in the nontreated group and 8 in the treated group. This difference, however, was not significant. Information about the clinical presentation and impact of symptomatic episodes was not provided, and the clinical significance of the potential decrease in symptomatic episodes is difficult to assess. If there is a benefit of treatment of asymptomatic bacteriuria in elderly ambulant women, there would also be an argument for screening for bacteriuria in this population. Such an approach does not seem rational given the current limited evidence for short- or long-term morbidity and the high prevalence of bacteriuria (62).

One prospective descriptive study in ambulatory elderly men addressed the question of the potential impact of treatment of asymptomatic bacteriuria (63). The majority (76%) of 29 elderly men identified with bacteriuria on screening cultures had spontaneous resolution of bacteriuria. During 1 to 4.5 years follow-up, only 5 episodes of symptomatic infection occurred in these 29, and no episodes in 104 other elderly men who did not develop asymptomatic bacteriuria. The authors concluded there was no evidence to support screening for or treatment of asymptomatic bacteriuria in ambulatory elderly men.

Fifty highly functionally impaired elderly women permanently resident in a long-term care facility with asymptomatic bacteriuria were randomized to therapy or no therapy and followed for 12 months (15). The overall prevalence of bacteriuria was decreased by approximately 30% in those who received intensive antimicrobial therapy for all episodes of bacteriuria during the follow-up period. The occurrence of symptomatic urinary infection was similar for treated or nontreated groups. Women treated for asymptomatic bacteriuria had a significantly increased frequency of reinfection with resistant organisms and adverse drug effects. Survival was similar for the treated and nontreated groups. Thus, treatment of asymptomatic bacteriuria in elderly institutionalized women is not beneficial, and may be harmful.

Another study in 36 functionally impaired institutionalized elderly men randomized to therapy or no therapy and followed for 2 years reported that all subjects who survived for 2 years remained bacteriuric at the end of the trial, despite intensive interval antimicrobial therapy in the treatment group (14). The prevalence of bacteriuria decreased in the treated group, with 56% of those randomized to therapy bacteriuric for over half the 24 study months as compared with 100% of those randomized to no therapy. Episodes of infectious morbidity, including symptomatic urinary infection and mortality, were similar for the two groups. Thus, no benefits of treatment of asymptomatic bacteriuria in these men were identified.

One consistent observation in institutionalized populations is the extraordinary frequency of recurrent infection following antimicrobial therapy (14,15). Over half of women have recurrence within 4 weeks of antimicrobial therapy (64). Most men ultimately have recurrent infection, although some may have prolonged periods free of bacteriuria (14). Thus, efforts to treat asymptomatic bacteriuria in the institutionalized population would require repeated antimicrobial therapy for a substantial proportion of residents. This would be associated with excess cost and adverse drug effects and would promote the emergence of resistant organisms. It has been suggested that pyuria with asymptomatic bacteriuria is an indication for therapy. However, as previously noted, over 90% of elderly subjects with asymptomatic bacteriuria have associated pyuria. There is no clinical evidence to suggest different outcomes with respect to mortality on the basis of quantitative differences in pyuria (65). Thus, a recommendation for treatment of asymptomatic bacteriuria if pyuria is also present is not currently justified.

Cranberry juice has also been reported to be beneficial for asymptomatic bacteriuria in the elderly (66). The benefit, however, was for a decreased frequency of bacteriuria with pyuria, not bacteriuria itself. In addition, cranberry juice intake did not lead to a decreased occurrence of symptomatic infection. Thus, while one would not discourage individuals from drinking large quantities of cranberry juice, current evidence is insufficient to suggest a clinical benefit.

Symptomatic Urinary Tract Infection

Antimicrobial Selection

Symptomatic urinary infection should, of course, be treated. The selection of antimicrobial does not differ substantively in the elderly as compared with a younger population. Many changes in antimicrobial pharmacokinetics occur with aging, including an increased volume of distribution for antimicrobials and aging-associated declines in creatinine clearance (67). These changes are not of a consistency or degree such that routine modification of agent or dose solely on the basis of age is recommended (67). As in any population, dosage will vary with renal function. Selected agents appropriate for treatment of urinary infection for which wide clinical experience is available are listed in Table 4.

Comparative clinical trials to evaluate efficacy and safety of different antimicrobials in the elderly are limited. The few studies reported (68–72) are compromised by small study numbers, failure to obtain long-term follow-up after therapy, and inclusion of asymptomatic subjects. It is difficult, then, to make statements about the comparative efficacy of an-

TABLE 4. *Antimicrobials useful in the treatment of urinary tract infection in the elderly*

Oral	Dosage[a]
amoxicillin[b]	500 mg tid
amoxicillin/clavulanic acid	500 mg tid
cephalexin	250–500 mg qid
ciprofloxacin	250–500 mg bid
nitrofurantoin[b]	50 mg qid
nitrofurantoin macrocrystals	100 mg qid
norfloxacin	400 mg bid
ofloxacin	400 mg od or bid
trimethoprim[b]	100 mg bid
trimethoprim/sulfamethoxazole[b]	160/800 mg bid
Parenteral	
amikacin	15 mg/kg/day q12h or q24h
ampicillin[b]	1 g q6h
cefazolin	1 g q8h
ceftriaxone	1 g q24h
cefotaxime	1 g q8h
ceftazidime	1 g q8h
ciprofloxacin	400 mg q12h
gentamicin[b]	5 mg/kg/day q12h or q24h
imipenem	500 mg q6h
tobramycin	5 mg/kg/day q12h or q24h
trimethoprim/sulfamethoxazole	160/800 mg bid
ticarcillin/clavulanate	50 mg/kg q6h

[a]For subjects with normal renal function.
[b]First-line agents.

timicrobials for treatment of urinary infection in the elderly. Selection of an agent for which there is wide clinical experience in the treatment of urinary infection, to which the infecting organism is known to be or likely to be susceptible, and that is tolerated by the patient is appropriate. When these factors are equivalent, cost, and, for long-term care institutions, potential to promote antimicrobial resistance may also be important considerations.

As a general rule, trimethoprim/sulfamethoxazole or nitrofurantoin would be considered as first-line therapy. Amoxicillin is preferred for gram-positive organisms. The fluoroquinolones should be reserved for patients intolerant to first-line agents or known or suspected to have resistant organisms. If parenteral therapy is required, ampicillin plus an aminoglycoside remains standard empiric therapy.

Urine cultures following therapy to document sterility are generally not indicated. Subjects will frequently be bacteriuric after therapy. Unless symptoms attributable to recurrent urinary infection are present, the presence or absence of bacteriuria after therapy is not clinically relevant.

The diagnostic uncertainty inherent in the institutionalized elderly compromises optimal antimicrobial use. While antimicrobial therapy is not appropriate for the treatment of chronic genitourinary symptoms, gross hematuria, malodorous urine, or nonspecific decline in status, the therapeutic decision in the individual patient may not be clear-cut. Thus, it may be necessary to treat for presumed or possible symptomatic urinary infection in a bacteriuric subject, although the clinical presentation is not straightforward. In this situation it would seem most appropriate to define the "symptoms" one is attempting to alter and review the patient after 48 to 72 hours to determine whether or not the antimicrobial has been effective. If there has been no response, it is probably not appropriate to persist with antimicrobial therapy.

Duration of Therapy

The optimal duration of therapy for urinary infection in the elderly has not been well studied. Studies in women consistently report a poorer outcome with any duration of therapy in postmenopausal as compared with younger women (73–75). Older women may have a particularly poor outcome with very short courses of therapy, such as a single dose or 3-day dosing (75,76). Elderly women with symptomatic lower urinary tract infection should likely receive a 7-day course of therapy. Further comparative studies of duration of therapy in this population are needed. For women with invasive urinary infection, usually manifesting as pyelonephritis, an initial 2-week course of therapy is recommended.

The duration of therapy for men with symptomatic urinary infection is complicated by the high frequency of prostatic infection. As stated earlier, prostatic infection is difficult or impossible to eradicate. If present, it generally warrants more prolonged courses of therapy. For acute symptomatic urinary infection in male patients, an appropriate initial duration of therapy is 2 weeks. If symptomatic relapse occurs, suggesting a prostatic source, retreatment with 6 or 12 weeks of therapy is indicated (77,78).

Long-Term Antimicrobial Therapy

Prolonged antimicrobial use for urinary infection in elderly populations should be considered in only highly selected clinical situations. In the institutionalized population in particular, the potential for long term-antimicrobial therapy to lead to antimicrobial resistance must be considered.

There are two instances in which there is a role for long-term therapy. The first is recurrent symptomatic cystitis in elderly women. Studies of long-term, low-dose antimicrobial prophylaxis for the prevention of recurrent cystitis specific to elderly women have not been published, but older women have been enrolled in many reported studies (79). These have not reported a differential response in postmenopausal as compared with younger women. The most appropriate regimens are trimethoprim/sulfamethoxazole tablet at bedtime daily or 3 times weekly, trimethoprim 100 mg at bedtime, or nitrofurantoin 50 or 100 mg at bedtime. Norfloxacin 200 mg daily and cephalexin 250 mg daily are also effective but are second-line choices owing to cost or limited experience. Topical vaginal estrogen therapy may provide a nonantimicrobial option for infection prevention for selected postmenopausal women, but further study of this approach as compared with antimicrobial therapy is needed (27).

Men with relapsing infection from a prostatic focus may require long-term suppressive therapy to prevent symptomatic recurrences (80). Men or women may experience recurrent episodes of invasive urinary infection in the presence of underlying abnormalities associated with obstruction, such as stones, tumors, or strictures. If the genitourinary abnormality cannot be surgically corrected, long-term suppressive therapy may be necessary to prevent invasive infection or struvite stone enlargement. The antimicrobial selected for suppressive therapy would be determined by the susceptibilities of the organism isolated from the urine. Therapy is usually started at full therapeutic doses, and may be decreased to about half the initial dose once the patient is stable and the urine culture is negative.

REFERENCES

1. Kemper P, Murtaugh CM. Lifetime use of nursing home care. *N Engl J Med* 1991;324:595.
2. Nicolle LE. Topics in long term care: urinary tract infections in long-term care facilities. *Infect Control Hosp Epidemiol* 1993;14:220.
3. Warren JW. Catheter-associated urinary tract infections. *Infect Dis Clin North Am* 1987;1:823.
4. Nicolle LE. Prevention and treatment of urinary catheter related infections in older patients. *Drugs Aging* 1994;4:379.
5. Boscia JA, Kobasa WD, Knight RA. Epidemiology of bacteriuria in an elderly ambulatory population. *Am J Med* 1986;80:208.
6. Sourander LB. Urinary tract infection in the aged. *Ann Med Intern Fenn* 1966;55(Suppl 45):7.
7. Brocklehurst JC, Dillane JB, Griffiths L, Fry J. The prevalence and symptomatology of urinary infection in an aged population. *Gerontol Clin* 1968;10:242.
8. Akhtar AJ, Andrew GR, Caird TI, Fallon RJ. Urinary tract infection in the elderly: A population study. *Age Ageing* 1972;1:48.
9. Nordenstam GR, Branberg CA, Oden AS, Svanborg-Eden CM, Svanborg A. Bacteriuria and mortality in an elderly population. *N Engl J Med* 1986;314:1152.
10. Abrutyn E, Mossey J, Levison M, Boscia J, Pitsakis P, Kaye D. Epidemiology of asymptomatic bacteriuria in elderly women. *J Am Geriatr Soc* 1991;39:388.
11. Wolfson SA, Kalmanson GM, Rubini ME, Guze LB. Epidemiology of bacteriuria in a predominantly geriatric male population. *Am J Med Sci* 1965;87:168.
12. Gladstone JL, Friedman SA. Bacteriuria in the aged: a study of its prevalence and predispoing lesions in a chronically ill population. *J Urol* 1971;106:745.
13. Kasviki-Charvati P, Drolette-Kefakis B, Papanayiatou PC, Dontas AS. Turnover of bacteriuria in old age. *Age Ageing* 1982;11:169.
14. Nicolle LE, Bjornson J, Harding GKM, MacDonell JA. Bacteriuria in elderly institutionalized men. *N Engl J Med* 1983;309:142.
15. Nicolle LE, Mayhew WJ, Bryan L. Prospective randomized comparison of therapy and no therapy for asymptomatic bacteriuria in institutionalized elderly women. *Am J Med* 1987;83:27.

16. Bentzen A, Vejlsgaard R. Asymptomatic bacteriuria in elderly subjects. *Dan Med Bull* 1980;27:101.
17. Walkey FA, Judge TG, Thompson J, Sarkari NBS. Incidence of urinary infection in the elderly. *Scott Med J* 12:411, 1967.
18. Gaynes RP, Weinstein RA, Chamberlin W, Kabins SA. Antibiotic resistant flora in nursing home patients admitted to the hospital. *Arch Intern Med* 1985;145:1804.
19. Gleckman R, Blagg N, Hibert D. Community-acquired bacteremic urosepsis in elderly patients: a prospective study of 34 consecutive episodes. *J Urol* 1983;128:79.
20. Gleckman RA, Bradley PJ, Roth RM, Hibert DM. Bacteremic urosepsis: a phenomenon unique to elderly women. *J Urol* 1985;133:174.
21. Muder RR, Brennen C, Wagener MM, Goetz AM. Bacteremia in a long-term care facility: a five year prospective study of 163 consecutive episodes. *Clin Infect Dis* 1992;14:647.
22. Senay H, Getz MB. Epidemiology of bacteremic urinary tract infections in chronically hospitalized elderly men. *J Urol* 1991;145:1201.
23. Nicolle LE, McIntyre M, Hoban D, Murray D. Bacteremia in a long term care facility. *Can J Infect Dis* 1994;5:130.
24. Gleckman R, Esposito A, Crowley M, Natsios GA. Reliability of single urine culture in establishing diagnosis of asymptomatic bacteriuria in adults males. *J Clin Microbiol* 1979;9:596.
25. Ouslander JG, Greengold BA, Silverblatt FJ, Garcia JP. An accurate method to obtain urine for culture in men with external catheters. *Arch Intern Med* 1987;147:286.
26. Nicolle LE, Harding GKM, Kennedy J, McIntyre M, Aoki F, Murray D. Urine specimen collection with external devices for diagnosis of bacteriuria in elderly incontinent men. *J Clin Microbiol* 1988;26:1115.
27. Raz R, Stamm WE. A controlled trial of intravaginal estriol in post-menopausal women with recurrent urinary tract infections. *New Engl J Med* 1993;329:753.
28. Stamey TA, Fair WR, Timothy MM, et al. Antibacterial nature of prostatic fluid. *Nature* 1968;218:444.
29. Hirsh DD, Fainstein V, Musher DM. Do condom catheter collecting systems cause urinary tract infection? *JAMA* 1979;242:340.
30. Suntharalingan M, Seth V, Moore-Smith B. Site of urinary tract infection in elderly women admitted to an acute geriatric assessment unit. *Age Ageing* 1983;12:317.
31. Nicolle LE, Muir P, Harding GKM, Norris M. Localization of site of urinary infection in elderly institutionalized women with asymptomatic bacteriuria. *J Infect Dis* 1988; 157:65.
32. Svanborg-Eden C, de Man P. Bacterial virulence in urinary tract infection. *Infect Dis Clin North Am* 1987;1:731.
33. Nicolle LE, Norris M, Finlayson M. Hemagglutination characteristics of Escherichia coli isolates from elderly women with asymptomatic bacteriuria. In: Kass EH, Svanborg-Eden C, eds. *Host-parasite interactions in urinary tract infections.* Chicago: University of Chicago Press; 1989:62–65.
34. Rodgers K, Nicolle LE, McIntyre M, Harding GKM, Hoban D, Murray D. Pyuria in institutionalized elderly subjects. *Can J Infect Dis* 1991;2:142.
35. Boscia JA, Abrutyn E, Levison ME, Pitsakis PG, Kaye D. Pyuria and asymptomatic bacteriuria in elderly ambulatory women. *Ann Intern Med* 1989;110:404.
36. Nicolle LE, Brunka J. Urinary IgG and IgA antibodies in elderly institutionalized subjects with bacteriuria. *Gerontology* 1990;36:345.
37. Nicolle LE, Brunka J, Orr P, Wilkins J, Harding GKM. Urinary immunoreactive interleukin-1 alpha and interleukin-6 in bacteriuric institutionalized elderly subjects. *J Urol* 1993;149:1049.
38. Nicolle LE, Brunka J, Ujack E, Bryan L. Antibodies to major outer membrane proteins of Escherichia coli in urinary infection in the elderly. *J Infect Dis* 1989;160:627.
39. Irvine PW, van Buren M, Crossley K. Causes of hospitalization of nursing home residents: the role of infection. *J Amer Ger Soc* 1984;32:103.
40. Boscia JA, Kobasa WD, Knight RA, Abrutyn E, Levison ME, Kaye D. Therapy vs no therapy for bacteriuria in elderly ambulatory non-hospitalized women. *J Amer Med Assoc* 1987;257:1067.
41. Carty M, Brocklehurst JC, Carty J. Bacteriuria and its correlates in old age. *Gerontology* 1981;27:72.

42. Boscia JA, Kobasa WD, Abrutyn E, Levison ME, Kaplan AM, Kaye D. Lack of association between bacteriuria and symptoms in the elderly. *Am J Med* 1986;81:979.
43. Berman P, Hogan DB, Fox RA. The atypical presentation of infection in old age. *Age Ageing* 1987;16:201.
44. Nicolle LE, McIntyre M, Zacharias H, MacDonell JA. Twelve month surveillance of infections in institutionalized elderly men. *J Am Geriatr Soc* 1984;32:513.
45. Garibaldi R, Brodine S, Matsumiya R. Infections among patients in nursing homes: policies, prevalence, and problems. *New Engl J Med* 1981;305:731–735.
46. Gordon WZ, Kane RL, Rothenberg R. Acute hospitalization in a home for the aged. *J Am Geriatr Soc* 1984;33:519.
47. Orr PH, Nicolle LE, Duckworth H, et al. Fever in the institutionalized elderly. *31st Conference on Antimicrobial Agents and Chemotherapy.* Chicago, 1991:Abstract No. 934.
48. Siroky MB, Maylan RA, Austen G, Olsson CA. Metastatic infection secondary to genitourinary tract sepsis. *Am J Med* 1976;63:351.
49. Nicolle LE, Orr P, Duckworth H, et al. Gross hematuria in residents of long term care facilities. *Am J Med* 1993;94:611.
50. Nicolle LE. Consequences of asymptomatic bacteriuria in the elderly. *Int J Antimicrob Agents* 1994;4:107.
51. Nicolle LE, Orr P, Duckworth H, et al. Prospective study of decubitus ulcers in two long term care facilities. *Can J Infect Control* 1994;9:35.
52. Dontas AS, Kasviki-Charvati P, Papanayiotou PC, Marketos SG. Bacteriuria and survival in old age. *N Engl J Med* 1981;304:939.
53. Sourander LB, Dasanen A. A five-year follow-up of bacteriuria in the aged. *Gerontol Clin* (Basel) 1972;14:274.
54. Heinamaki P, Haavisto M, Hakullnen T, Mattela K, Rajala S. Mortality in relation to urinary characteristics in the very aged. *Gerontology* 1986;32:167.
55. Nicolle LE, Henderson E, Bjornson J, McIntyre M, Harding GKM, MacDonell JA. The association of bacteriuria with resident characteristics and survival in elderly institutionalized men. *Ann Intern Med* 1987;106:682.
56. Abrutyn E, Mossey J, Berlin JA, et al. Does asymptomatic bacteriuria predict mortality and does antimicrobial treatment reduce mortality in elderly ambulatory women. *Ann Intern Med* 1994;120:827.
57. Kohn RR. Cause of death in very old people. *JAMA* 1982;247;2793.
58. Puxty JAH, Horan MA, Fox RA. Necropses in the elderly. *Lancet* 1983;1:1262.
59. Crossley K, Henry K, Irvine P, et al. Antibiotic use in nursing homes: prevalence, cost, and utilization review. *Bull NY Acad Med* 1987;63:510.
60. Warren JW, Palumbo FB, Fitterman L, Speedie SM. Incidence and characteristics of antibiotics in aged nursing home patients. *J Am Geriatr Soc* 1991;39:963.
61. Zimmer JG, Bentley DW, Valenti WM, Watson NM. Systemic antibiotic use in nursing homes. A quality assessment. *J Am Geriatr Soc* 1986;34:703.
62. Canadian Task Force on the Periodic Health Examination Screening for Asymptomatic Bacteriuria in the Elderly. *The Canadian guide to clinical preventive health care.* Ottawa: Health Canada; 1994:966–974.
63. Mims AD, Norman DC, Yamamura RH, Yoshikawa TT. Clinically inapparent (asymptomatic) bacteriuria in ambulatory elderly men. Epidemiological, clinical, and microbiological findings. *J Am Geriatr Soc* 1990;38:1209.
64. Nicolle LE, Mayhew JW, Bryan L. Outcome following antimicrobial therapy for asymptomatic bacteriuria in elderly women resident in an institution. *Age Ageing* 1988;17:187.
65. Nicolle LE, Brunka J, McIntyre M, Murray D, Harding GKM. Asymptomatic bacteriuria, urinary antibody, and survival in the institutionalized elderly. *J Am Geriatr Soc* 1992;40:607.
66. Avorn J, Monane M, Gurwitz JH, Glynn RJ, Choodnovskiy J, Lipsitz LA. Reduction of bacteriuria and pyuria after ingestion of cranberry juice. *JAMA* 1994 271:751.
67. Ljunberg B, Nilsson-Ehle I. Pharmacokinetics of antimicrobial agents in the elderly. *Rev Infect Dis* 1987;9:250.
68. Leigh DA, Smith EC, Marrimer J. Comparative study using norfloxacin and amoxicillin in the treatment of complicated urinary tract infections in geriatric patients. *J Antimicrob Chemother* 1984;13(Suppl B):79.

69. Hill S, Yeates M, Pathy J, Morgan JR. A controlled trial of norfloxacin and amoxicillin in the treatment of uncomplicated urinary tract infection in the elderly. *J Antimicrob Chemother* 1985;15:505.
70. Ewer TC, Bailey RR, Gilchrist NL, Aitken JM, Sainsburg R. Comparative study of norfloxacin and trimethoprim for the treatment of elderly patients with urinary tract infection. *NZ Med J* 1988;101:537.
71. Tzias V, Dontas AS, Petrikkos G, Papapetropoulou M, Dracopoulos J, Giamarellou H. Three-day antibiotic therapy in bacteriuria of old age. *J Antimicrob Chemother* 1990;26:705.
72. Giamarellou H, Iakovou M, Pistoni M, Petrikkas G, Dontas A, Sfikakis P. Kinetics and comparative efficacy of ofloxacin versus cotrimoxazole in the asymptomatic bacteriuria of elderly subjects. *Chemotherapy* 1991;37(Suppl 1):19.
73. Cardenas J, Quinn EL, Roober G, Gavinger J, Pohlod D. Single-dose cephalexin therapy for acute bacterial urinary tract infections and acute urethral syndrome with bladder bacteriuria. *Antimicrob Agents Chemother* 1986;29:383.
74. Harding GKM, Nicolle LE, Ronald AR, *et al.* Management of catheter acquired urinary tract infection in women: therapy following catheter removal. *Ann Intern Med* 1991;114:713.
75. Saginur R, Nicolle LE, Canadian Infectious Diseases Society Clinical Trials Group. Single dose of three days norfloxacin for acute uncomplicated urinary infection in women. *Arch Intern Med* 1992;152:1233.
76. Flanagan PG, Rooney PJ, Davies EA, Stout RW. A comparison of single-dose versus conventional-dose antibiotic treatment of bacteriuria in elderly women. *Age Ageing* 1991;20:206.
77. Gleckman R, Crowley M, Natsios GA. Therapy for recurrent invasive urinary tract infections in men. *N Engl J Med* 1979;301:878.
78. Smith JW, Jones SR, Reed WP, Tice AD, Deupree RH, Kaiser B. Recurrent urinary tract infections in men: characteristics and response to therapy. *Ann Intern Med* 1979;91:544.
79. Nicolle LE, Ronald AR. Recurrent urinary tract infection in adult women: diagnosis and treatment. *Infect Dis Clin North Am* 1987;1:793.
80. Freeman RB, Smith WM, Richardson JA, et al. Long term therapy for chronic bacteriuria in men: US Public Health Service cooperative study. *Ann Intern Med* 1975;83:133.

Antibiotic Therapy in Urology,
edited by S. Grant Mulholland, M.D.,
Lippincott-Raven Publishers, Philadelphia © 1996.

Chapter 5

Prostatitis

J. Curtis Nickel

Department of Urology, Queen's University, Kingston, Ontario, K7L 2V7 Canada

INTRODUCTION

The management of the various prostatitis syndromes remains a problem for the practicing clinical urologist in the 1990s. Although it was recognized in the 1930s (1) that prostatitis could be caused by bacteria in the prostate gland, it was not until 1968 that Meares and Stamey (2) described a standardized bacteriologic localization procedure for men with prostatitis syndromes. A clinically relevant classification system (3) based on this rigid bacteriologic diagnosis system has now become accepted by most researchers and practicing physicians (Table 1). Subsequent research in antibiotic pharmacokinetics in the prostate gland led to further insights into treatment (4). It would seem reasonable, then, that with an understanding of the etiology of the various syndromes, a standardized method of classification based on a rigorous diagnostic system, and knowledge of the pharmacokinetics of antibiotics in the prostate that the treatment of prostatitis should not be a problem. In reality, the etiologic basis of the various disease processes is poorly understood, the clinical presentation is extremely variable, the diagnosis is difficult, especially in previously treated patients, and treatment regimes are not always successful, even in patients with a bacteriologically proven prostatic infection. Frustration and confusion by both physicians and patients still surround this clinical entity. In the 1980s prostatitis was described as a continuing enigma (5), which continues into the 1990s (6).

ETIOLOGY AND PATHOGENESIS

The etiology and pathogenesis of the various prostatitis syndromes are complicated by the fact that although the clinical symptomatology can be very similar, the etiologic bases of bacterial and nonbacterial prostatitis and prostatodynia (which is not really prostatic inflammation at all) are quite different (6). Some facts regarding the etiology of bacterial pro-

TABLE 1. *The prostatitis syndromes*

Acute bacterial prostatitis	
	Acute inflammation of the prostate gland is characterized by leukocytosis in the prostatic fluid and positive bacterial cultures of the prostatic fluid (if obtained), bladder urine (usually), and blood (occasionally).
Chronic bacterial prostatitis	
	Chronic bacterial inflammation of the prostate gland is characterized by leukocytosis and positive bacterial cultures in the prostatic fluid but rarely in the bladder urine.
Nonbacterial prostatitis	
	Chronic inflammation of the prostate gland is characterized by leukocytosis of the prostatic fluid but no positive bladder or prostatic cultures of the "usual" bacterial pathogens.
Prostatodynia[a]	
	Prostate demonstrates no inflammation and cultures are all sterile.

[a]The author suggests that prostatodynia be dropped from the prostatitis classification system, renamed as "pelvic floor myalgia," and relegated to an important role in the differential diagnosis. Rationale for this modification to our standard classification system is presented in the text.

statitis are generally accepted. The bacteria causing both acute and chronic bacterial prostatitis are similar in type and incidence to those that cause simple urinary tract infections (UTIs), with aerobic gram-negative enteric bacteria (especially *Escherichia coli*) being the most common (7,8). The role of gram-positive bacteria is unclear, although many accept that enterococci can be an etiologic agent (9). Great controversy exists as to whether or not other gram-positive bacteria, such as coagulase-negative staphylococci, are causative organisms in prostatitis (10). Anaerobic bacteria have also been isolated in the prostatic secretion; however it remains uncertain whether these are responsible for the prostatic inflammation.

The etiologic organism (if there is in fact an organism) in nonbacterial prostatitis remains elusive. *Ureaplasma* and/or *Chlamydia* have been proposed as possible etiologic organisms. The results of recent research in the role of these organisms as etiologic agents in nonbacterial prostatitis remain extremely conflicting (11–16). Any critical analysis of the literature would have to conclude that we don't have the answer and clinicians should consider these organisms as only potential etiologic agents in this disease. Coagulase-negative staphylococci, which are dismissed by many researchers and clinicians as only urethral contaminants, may in fact be implicated in low-grade inflammation of the prostate gland (8,10,17); therefore some patients who have been given a diagnosis of nonbacterial prostatitis may in fact have a bacterial prostatitis caused by one of these seemingly innocuous organisms. Alternatively, these organisms may be only innocent bystanders in the inflammatory process. Patients with chronic bacterial prostatitis who remain clinically refractory to antibiotic therapy, even with a supposed bacteriologic cure, may continue to have symptoms. This may be because of the persistent presence of bacteria or retained bacterial antigens in the prostate gland that have become difficult or even impossible to demonstrate using standard culture techniques (18). Such patients could be improperly classified as having nonbacterial prostatitis, primarily because the diagnostic techniques were done after treatment was instituted. However, none of these agents may be implicated in a great percentage of patients with nonbacterial prostatic inflammation. It has been hypothesized that the inflammation may be related to intraprostatic reflux of sterile urine (19), causing nonspecific areas of chronic inflammation (20). This nonspecific inflammation may have an immunologic basis (20,21).

No infectious agent can be localized in quantitative cultures and there is no inflammatory response in the prostatic secretions of patients with prostatodynia (22). The prostate gland does not seem to be involved in the clinical symptomatology at all (23). The etiology remains elusive, but it appears to involve a neuromuscular dysfunction of the pelvic floor or perineum.

The etiologic agents in this disease remain confusing, and the pathophysiology is even more so. It appears that the bacteria enter the prostate gland from the urethra, perhaps assisted by turbulent urethral flow patterns and/or intraprostatic ductal reflux (6,24,25,26). Animal modeling of prostatitis (27,28,29), supported by clinical studies involving that difficult group of patients with bacterial prostatitis that remains refractory to therapy (18), has led to a further understanding of what is actually happening in the prostate gland during acute and then chronic bacterial prostatitis. Once the bacteria enter the ducts and acini of the prostate gland, they rapidly multiply, inducing a host response with infiltration of acute inflammatory cells into the ducts. In acute bacterial prostatitis, the entire prostate gland or at least the major part of it is involved in the inflammatory process. The ducts become engorged with infiltrate made up of dead and live bacteria as well as living and dying acute inflammatory cells, desquamated epithelial cells, and cellular debris. At this point it is relatively easy to eradicate all the offending organisms with appropriate antibiotic therapy for complete resolution of the inflammatory process. If bacteria persist from either acute or, more likely, clinically subacute inflammation, they can form small, sporadic microcolonies within the ductal system adherent to the epithelium (Fig. 1).

The bacteria produce an exopolysaccharide slime or glycocalyx that envelops these microcolonies, and the microorganisms subsequently become very quiescent, undergoing a sort of "hibernation" when the environment becomes threatening. Surrounding these focal sites of bacterial persistence are areas of lymphocytic invasion with variable infiltration of plasma cells and macrophages. It appears that the bacteria persisting in the prostate gland in these focal areas or alternatively reinfections of the prostate gland by similar bacteria lead to persistent immunologic stim-

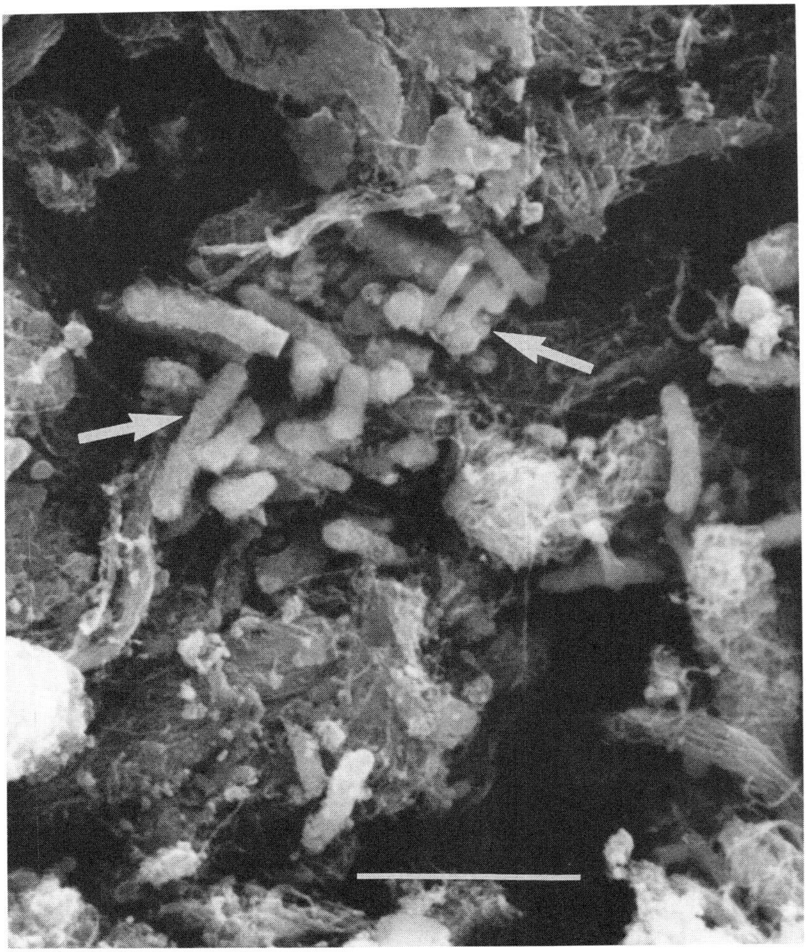

FIG. 1. Scanning electron micrograph of a bacterial microcolony or small biofilm (*arrows*) adherent to a prostatic duct in a patient with a 2-year clinical history of initially documented *Escherichia coli* chronic prostatitis. At the time of biopsy the patient had not been taking antibiotics for a period of 4 weeks. Expressed prostatic fluid was sterile, but culture of transperineal needle biopsies of the prostate revealed *E. coli.* (Magnification bar = 5 μ) (Electron photomicrograph from the author's ongoing prostatitis studies. Magnification bar, 5 μ.)

ulation. The subsequent focal inflammation is the body's attempt to eradicate the persistent bacterial microcolonies. Over time fibrosis occurs with subsequent permanent scarring.

The prostatic inflammation that develops in patients with nonbacterial prostatitis is confusing. The noted deposition of antibody and complement in the focal areas of inflammation (20) may be caused by undetected organisms or represent a reaction to either refluxing urine or urine toxins (19,21).

It becomes clear therefore that except for somewhat rare cases of proven bacterial prostatitis supported by our presently available diagnostic tests, the etiology in the vast majority of patients presenting with prostatitis symptoms remains confusing.

DIAGNOSIS

The history and physical examination may suggest the diagnosis, but most signs and symptoms of bacterial prostatitis, nonbacterial prostatitis, and even prostatodynia remain indistinguishable (30). The familiar but difficult, time-consuming, and even expensive diagnostic routine remains the accepted key to diagnosis (31). Excessive leukocytosis in a smear of the expressed prostatic secretion (EPS) remains helpful, but the gold standard for diagnosis of a bacterial etiology of chronic prostatitis symptoms remains the specific-culture technique as described by Meares and Stamey (2) 25 years ago.

Most urologists have a working understanding of the rationale, methodology, and interpretation of the simultaneous quantitative bacterial cultures of urethral and bladder urine and EPS (Fig. 2). A definitive diagnosis of chronic bacterial prostatitis is confirmed when a quantitative

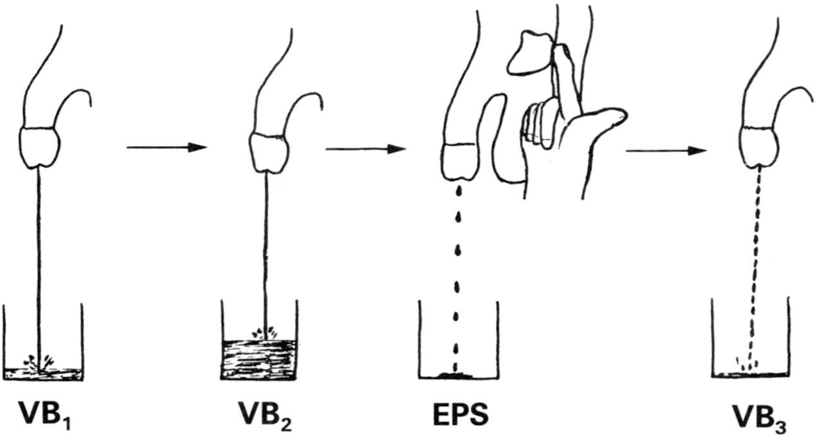

FIG. 2. Segmented cultures of the lower urinary tract in men. This technique is based on sequential collections of a urethral specimen (initially voided urine or VB1), bladder specimen (midstream urine or VB2), and prostatic specimens (expressed prostatic secretion or EPS, and urine voided immediately after massage or VB3). The problems with this diagnostic scheme and the reasons why it has largely been abandoned by most family physicians and urologists are outlined in the text.

bacterial count demonstrates a significantly higher number of bacteria per milliliter in the EPS (or voided urine after prostatic massage—VB3) compared with that in VB1 (first voided urine) or VB2 (midstream urine) specimens. The original report of this technique included only five patients, was not properly controlled, and in fact has never been validated (2). The majority of practicing urologists do not use this sequential culture technique. Informal polling of urologists at national and international meetings reveals that fewer than 5% routinely subject their patients with suspected prostatitis to these diagnostic techniques (26). The identifiable shortcomings or problems with our standardized diagnostic techniques include the following (32):

1. Prostatic secretion cannot be obtained from all patients all the time, and the postprostatic specimen (VB3) or ejaculate culture can be difficult to interpret.
2. Previous antibiotic therapy has invariably been prescribed by the primary physician without first obtaining the proper specimens, and this may mask subsequent attempts at bacterial localization.
3. The bacteria are firmly adherent to the ductal epithelium and may not be shed in significant numbers into the expressed prostatic fluid. This fact is recently understood.
4. Patients with identified bacterial prostatitis may not respond clinically to appropriate antibiotic therapy although a so-called "bacteriologic cure" may be obtained.
5. There are some patients with excessive leukocytosis in the expressed prostatic secretion but no significant bacteria present who have significantly benefited and even been cured clinically by antibiotic therapy.
6. The clinical relapses of previously proven cases of bacterial prostatitis are not always associated with a positive EPS culture.
7. As described in the original article, experience has confirmed that urethritis is diagnosed only in patients with easily diagnosed clinical urethritis (urethral discharge and local urethral symptoms).
8. The test to differentiate bacterial cystitis from prostatitis (since they often coexist on first presentation) is difficult to use.
9. These very difficult procedures are time-consuming and expensive and consistently provide an extremely low yield.

In 12 of 20 patients undergoing biopsy with a previous history of documented bacterial prostatitis that had become clinically refractory to therapy even with a presumed "bacteriologic cure" (negative EPS), the original organism noted prior to antibiotic therapy was cultured on a biopsy specimen (18). Positive cultures therefore in our standardized diagnostic test may point to a bacterial etiology; however, negative EPS cultures cannot rule out a bacterial pathogen. Even when gram-positive organisms are definitely localized to the EPS, controversy remains whether these organisms are etiologic agents or just contaminants. It has been consistently demonstrated that 30–40% of prostatitis patients respond to antibiotic therapy despite negative culture results (32,33,34). It remains clear to many that our current diagnostic methods, while remaining the best we have available, continue to pose a problem.

TREATMENT

Treatment of acute bacterial prostatitis does not pose a problem. Patients invariably respond quickly to empiric antibiotic therapy (initially parenteral in some cases, followed by pathogen-specific antibiotics). Chronic bacterial prostatitis on the other hand is much more difficult to treat. The answer to our therapeutic dilemma appeared to reside in a series of exciting and elaborate experiments reported over the past two decades on the diffusion of various antimicrobial agents from plasma into prostatic fluids (4).

A large number of pharmacokinetic studies were done on various canine models quantitating antimicrobial drug diffusion, and from these particular types of studies a number of antibiotics (trimethoprim, erythromycin, quinolones) have been described as the most suitable drugs for the treatment of prostatitis. This is based on the realization that only the non-ionized portion of the drug is lipid-soluble (which is required for drug transport across the human lipid membranes such as prostatic epithelium); therefore the dissociation constant of the drug is important in diffusion when the pH values of the plasma and prostatic fluid differ significantly. Unfortunately, however, pH relationships in human patients with chronic bacterial prostatitis appear to be significantly different from those described in dogs without prostatic inflammation (35,36). Human pharmacokinetic studies have also been criticized because analyzed prostatic fluid obtained by prostatic massage or ejaculate following oral or parenteral administration of the various antibiotics appears to be contaminated with seminal fluid or urine containing high concentrations of antibiotics. Homogenized human prostatectomy specimens have also been analyzed for drug content following preoperative antibiotic loading, but it is apparent that this method does not measure the concentration in the prostatic duct, particularly the inflamed duct. Notwithstanding all the theoretical pharmacokinetic data, trimethoprim/sulfamethoxazole (37) and more recently the new quinolones have the best-confirmed cure rates in reported prospective studies (38,39,40). Antibiotics cure documented chronic bacterial prostatitis in about 50% of patients in most reported series.

The long-term cure rate (several years) may be considerably less than that reported for short-term studies, and the actual relapse rate following antibiotic treatment of chronic prostatitis is unknown (32). While higher cure rates have been reported (as high as 80–90% with some quinolones), many of us who have taken part in such trials suspect that these rates are of bacterial eradication from the EPS only and also do not take into account those patients who relapse after the trial period is completed (usually less than 6 months). Bacteriologic cures, in which the offending bacteria are eliminated from the EPS but the patient continues to have symptoms or suffers clinical relapses, continue to be a major problem for the practicing urologist.

Why don't antibiotics cure chronic bacterial prostatitis more consistently? The reason does not appear to be the development of bacterial resistance to the antibiotic or antibiotic levels within the prostate (41) but rather the persistence of "hibernating" bacterial microcolonies or biofilms adherent to the ducts or within the corpora amylacea or prostatic calculi within the prostate (6,18,26,28,41).

Since the etiology for nonbacterial prostatitis remains unclear, it is even more difficult to recommend definitive curative therapy for this entity. The use of minocycline, doxycycline, or erythromycin in patients with clinical prostatic inflammation but negative EPS cultures appears warranted (but not substantiated by reported clinical series). In most cases the inflammation is probably not caused by a defined etiologic microorganism but is the response to some nonspecific inflammatory stimulus, so empiric antibiotic therapy will not be beneficial. Antibiotic therapy, however, may be therapeutic in those patients in whom the standard diagnostic tests have failed to disclose bacterial organisms for the reasons outlined in the section on diagnosis.

Even less is known about prostatodynia, except that antibiotics provide no benefit at all. Pharmacologic management of detrusor-sphincter dyssynergia may be improved with alpha blockers. Antianxiolytics and muscle relaxants help some patients, and biofeedback technology has demonstrated improvements in the symptoms of some of these patients (author's unpublished data). Until this chronic symptomatology can be better defined, curative therapy may remain elusive.

DISCUSSION: POTENTIAL SOLUTIONS TO THE PROSTATITIS ENIGMA

It would be extremely satisfying at this stage to state that we do have the answer to all our problems with etiology, diagnosis, and treatment of the prostatitis syndromes, but unfortunately this is not the case. We do, however, have to continue to manage our patients with the best tools we have at our disposal, and we can use the information we already possess on etiology, the tools that we presently have for diagnosis, and the modalities that are available for therapy.

Research continues to probe the questions we have raised regarding the prostatitis syndromes, and exciting developments will transform our approach to our patients, it is hoped in this decade.

Good prospective clinical (26) and animal (29) studies, looking specifically at both etiology and pathogenesis, may unlock some of the mysteries that surround these syndromes. Immunologic diagnosis may eventually hold the key to the differentiation of bacterial and nonbacterial etiology of chronic prostatic inflammation. Preliminary studies employing a bacterial antigen mixture to determine antibody shed in the prostatic secretion and VB3 of patients in whom prostatitis had become difficult or impossible to diagnose using standard techniques shows early promise (42,43). Our research group is continuing to explore this diagnostic modality, as it appears to hold great promise for the future (multicenter Canadian trial in progress). Transrectal prostatic ultrasonography, which provides objective data on the topography of the prostate gland, initially appeared to hold promise, but the echo pattern of inflamed prostates are nonspecific, and there was no one feature diagnostic of this condition (44). Transrectal or transperineal biopsy, perhaps directed by transrectal ultrasonography, may be helpful in the diagnosis of prostatic abscesses, but because of the very focal nature of the chronic inflammation and bacterial prostatitis, it appears to be more a hit-and-miss technique that is not recommended except as a research tool at the present time (18).

Our standard classification of the prostatitis syndromes can now be modified because of our improved understanding of the pathogenesis of prostatic inflammation. Prostatodynia, which does not involve prostatic inflammation at all, can be ruled out by the absence of leukocytosis in EPS or the sediment of VB3 (32,42,43) and should be dropped from the classification system for prostatitis syndromes. Instead, it should more correctly be labeled as pelvic floor myalgia and be relegated to the role of an important differential diagnosis.

We must continue to use the standard sequential, quantitative culture technique for diagnosis but must remember that it is most effective at the time of initial presentation and becomes severely limited once any type of therapy has been instituted. We have recommended a simplified diagnostic technique employing only a preprostatic and postprostatic massage urine specimen (pre-M and post-M) in patients who do not have clinical urethritis. Leukocytosis seen in microscopy of the centrifuged sediment of the post-M specimen (> WBC/HPF or 1 log greater than in pre-M) suggests prostatic inflammation. Cultures of the two specimens are interpreted similarly to the standard Meares-Stamey technique (Table 2). This proposed technique suffers from many of the limitations of the classic 3-glass test, but it is simpler, cost-effective, and in our area generally accepted by urologists, casualty officers, and family physicians. This

TABLE 2. *Premassage (pre-M) and postmassage (post-M) test for prostatitis*

This simplified, cost- and time-effective diagnostic technique is suggested for patients with the clinical diagnosis of a chronic prostatitis syndrome and no clinical evidence of urethritis (rationale for this test explained in text).

Technique:

1. After adequate cleansing of the penis and with the foreskin retracted, have the patient provide a midstream urine specimen. Label this specimen pre-M.
2. Perform a digital rectal examination to assess the patient's prostate and vigorously massage the prostate from the periphery toward the midline.
3. Have the patient immediately provide another urine specimen (the first 10 ml only). Label this specimen post-M.
4. Send the two specimens for microscopy (resuspended postcentrifuged sediment) and quantitative culture.

Interpetation:

1. Leukocytosis in post-M specimen (> WBC/HPF or 1 log increase in WBC/HPF compared with pre-M test) suggests the diagnosis of prostatitis.
2. Significant bacteriuria in post-M specimen (defined as any bacteria if pre-M specimen sterile or colony count per milliliter 1 log greater compared with pre-M specimen) suggests bacterial prostatitis.
3. Significant bacteriuria in both pre-M and post-M specimens suggests bacterial prostatitis associated with bacterial cystitis. (If confirmation of bacterial prostatitis is required, repeat pre-M and post-M cultures after 3 days of nitrofurantoin therapy.)

technique, involving microscopy and culture with the addition of a simple immunologic diagnostic step (pre-M and post-M specimens being tested against a crude antigen mixture of pathogenic bacteria and chlamydia as previously described), is presently being tested and validated in a multicenter Canadian study (research in progress by author). Other diagnostic clues, such as previously documented episodes of acute prostatitis, recurrent cystitis in men with clinical symptoms of prostatitis, and even response to antibiotic therapy, continue to prove helpful in suggesting bacterial etiology in men in whom the standard diagnostic techniques have failed.

The development of new antibiotics (such as some of the newer quinolones) may hold more promise for the future, but studies to date have been small, poorly controlled, and short-term. Only through large, prospective, randomized, long-term clinical trials will we be able to determine the relative efficacy of the newer antibiotics in the prostatitis syndromes. Further understanding of the pathophysiology of this disease may lead to different dosing schedules and even routes of administration of antibiotics. In acute exacerbations of chronic prostatitis, the bacteria are shed more easily in the EPS and become more susceptible to antibiotic therapy, and it is therefore reasonable to treat patients with chronic resistant symptoms only at the time of acute symptomatic flare-ups. Pulse-dose therapy (i.e., high intermittent pulses of antibiotics) may have advantages in eliminating persistent bacterial biofilms within the prostate gland. Direct injection of antimicrobial agents into the prostate (45,46) or anal mucosa (47) have been reported to result in apparent success. This approach as well as high-pressure prostatic urethral injection of antibiotics continues to be explored by a number of research groups, including our own. Hyperthermia or thermal therapy may also be included as a possible treatment, particularly for prostatitis with a nonbacterial etiology (48). Only with a better understanding of prostatodynia through specific research will we be able to suggest any type of curative therapy for this chronic symptomatology.

The prostatitis syndromes will continue to be a problem for the physician and the patient since the etiology, diagnosis, and treatment remain unclear. However, the clinician who assumes responsibility for treating patients with prostatitis must develop an understanding and awareness of the evolving research into these related syndromes. The physician must be convinced that the correct diagnosis, particularly at first presentation, will allow therapeutic efforts to be directed at the proper disease process. Research continues in the prostatitis syndromes, and it is hoped that this will lead to more accurate diagnostic methods and better treatment regimes and eventually improve our therapy of the perplexing problem of prostatitis.

REFERENCES

1. Nickel AC. The bacteriology of chronic prostatitis and seminal vesiculitis and elective localization of the bacteria as isolated. *J Urol* 1930;24:343.
2. Meares EM Jr, Stamey TA. bacteriologic localization patterns in bacterial prostatitis and urethritis. *Invest Urol* 1968;5:492.
3. Drach GW, Meares EM Jr, Fair WR, Stamey TA. Classification of benign disease associated with prostatic pain: prostatitis or prostatodynia? *J Urol* 1978;120:266.
4. Sharer WV, Fair WR. The pharmacokinetics of antibiotic diffusion in chronic bacterial prostatitis. *Prostate* 1982;3:139.
5. Pfau A. Prostatitis: a continuing enigma. *Urol Clin North Am* 1986;13:695.
6. Nickel JC, Olson ME. Prostatitis: the enigma continues. *Contemp Urol* (Can) 1991;14:4.
7. Drach GW. Problems in diagnosis of bacterial prostatitis: gram-negative, gram-positive and mixed infection. *J Urol* 1974;4:630.
8. Meares EM. Prostatitis. *Med Clin North Am* 1991;75:405.
9. Drach GW. Prostatitis: man's hidden infection. *Urol Clin North Am* 1975;2:499.
10. Nickel JC, Costerton JW. Coagulase-negative Staphyloccus in chronic prostatitis. *J Urol* 1992;147:398.
11. Doble A, Thomas BJ, Walker MM, Harris JR, Witherow RD, Taylor-Robinson D. The role of Chlamydia trachomatis in chronic abacterial prostatitis: a study using ultrasound guided biopsy. *J Urol* 1989;14:332.
12. Bruce AW, Reid G. Prostatitis associated with Chlamydia trachomatis in 6 patients. *J Urol* 1989;142:1006.
13. Abelatif OMA, Chandler FW, McGuire BS. Chlamydia trachomatis in chronic abacterial prostatitis: demonstration by colorimetric in situ hybridization. *Hum Pathol* 1991;22:41.
14. Weidner W, Brunner H, Krause W. Quantitative culture of Ureaplasma urealyticum in patients with chronic prostatitis or prostatitis. *J Urol* 1980;124:622.
15. Brunner H, Weidner W, Shiefer HG. Studies on the role of Ureaplasma urealyticum and Mycoplasma hominis in prostatitis. *J Infect Dis* 1983;147:807.
16. Meares EM. Bacterial prostatitis vs "prostatosis": a clinical and bacteriological study. *JAMA* 1973;224:1372.
17. Wedren H. On chronic prostatitis with special studies of Staphylococcus epidermidis. *J Urol Nephrol* 1989;123(suppl):1.

18. Nickel JC, Costerton JW. Bacterial localization in antibiotic-refractory chronic bacterial prostatitis. *Prostate* 1993;23:107.
19. Kirby RS, Lowe D, Bultitude MI, Shuttleworth KED. Intraprostatic urinary reflux: an etiologic factor in abacterial prostatitis. *Br J Urol* 1982;54:729.
20. Doble A, Walker MM, Harris JRW, Taylor-Robinson D, Witherow RON. Intraprostatic antibody deposition in chronic abacterial prostatitis. *Br J Urol* 1991;65:598.
21. Keetch DW, Humphrey P, Ratliff TL. Development of a mouse model for nonbacterial prostatitis. *J Urol* 1994;152:247.
22. Barbalias GA, Meares EM Jr, Sant GR. Prostatodynia: clinical and urodynamic characteristics. *J Urol* 1983;130:514.
23. Barbalias GA. Prostatodynia or painful male urethral syndrome? *Urology* 1990;36:146.
24. Blacklock NJ. The anatomy of the prostate: relationship with prostatic inflammation. Infection 1991;19(Suppl 3):S111.
25. Nickel JC. A novel insight into the nature of chronic bacterial prostatitis. *J Urol* 1989;141:308A.
26. Nickel JC. New concepts in the pathogenesis and treatment of prostatitis. *Curr Opin Urol* 1992;2:37.
27. Nickel JC, Olson ME, Costerton JW. Rat model of experimental bacterial prostatitis. *Infection* 1991;19(suppl 3):S126.
28. Nickel JC, Olson ME, Barabas A, Benediktsson H, Dasgupta MK, Costerton JW. Pathogenesis of chronic bacterial prostatitis in an animal model. *Br J Urol* 1990;66:47.
29. Nickel JC, Olsen ME, Ceri H. Experimental prostatitis. In: Weidner W, Madson PO, Schiefer HG, eds. *Prostatitis: etiopathology, diagnosis and therapy.* Berlin: Springer-Verlag; 1994:123.
30. Nickel JC, The prostatitis syndromes. a continuing enigma for the family physician. *Can Fam Physician* 1991;37:921.
31. Nickel JC. Evaluation and management of the many syndromes in prostatitis. *Can J Diagnosis* 1989;6:19.
32. Nickel JC, Bruce AW, Reid G. Pathogenesis, diagnosis and treatment of the prostatitis syndromes. In: Krane KJ, Siroky MB, Fitzpatrick JM, eds. *Clinical urology.* Philadelphia: JB Lippincott; 1994:925.
33. Berger RE, Krieger JN, Kessler D, Ireton RC, Cose C, Homes KK, Roberts PL. Case control study of men with suspected chronic idiopathic prostatitis. *J Urol* 1989;141:328.
34. Weidner W, Schiefer HG, Kraus H, Jantos C, Friedrich HJ, Altmannsberger M. Chronic prostatitis: a thorough search for etiologically involved microoganisms in 1,461 patients. *Infection* 1991;19(Suppl 3):S119.
35. Fair WR, Crane DB, Schiller N, Heston WDW. Reappraisal of treatment in chronic bacterial prostatitis. *J Urol* 1979;121:437.
36. Pfau A, Perlberg S, Shapiro A. The pH of the prostatic fluid in health and disease: implications of treatment in chronic bacterial prostatitis. *J Urol* 1978;119:384.
37. Shaeffer AJ. Diagnosis and treatment of prostatitic infection. *Urol Suppl* 1990;36:13.
38. Naber KG. Use of quinolones in urinary tract infections and prostatitis. *Rev Infect Dis* 1989;11(suppl 5):S1321–S1337.
39. Aagaard J, Madsen PO. Bacterial prostatitis: new methods of treatment. *Urol Suppl* 1991;37:4.
40. Schaffer AJ, Dabras FS. The efficacy of norfloxacin in the treatment of chronic bacterial prostatitis refractory to trimethoprim-sulphamethoxazole and/or carbenicillin. *J Urol* 1990;144:690.
41. Nickel JC, Downey J, Clark J, Ceri H, Olson M. Antibiotic pharmacokinetics in the inflamed prostate. *J Urol* 1995;153:527–529.
42. Shortliffe LM, Elliott K, Sellers RG. Measurement of urinary antibodies to crude bacterial antigen in patients with chronic bacterial prostatitis. *J Urol* 1989;141:632.
43. Kumon H. Detection of a local prostatitis immune response to bacterial prostatitis. *Infection* 1992;20(Suppl 3):S236.
44. Doble A, Carter SS. Ultrasonographic findings in prostatitis. *Urol Clin North Am* 1989;16:763.
45. Jiminez-Cruz JF, Tormo FB, Gomez JG. Treatment of chronic prostatitis: intraprostatic antibiotic injections under echography control. *J Urol* 1988;139:967.

46. Baert L, Leonard A. Chronic bacterial prostatitis: 10 years experience with local antibiotic. *J Urol* 1988;140:755.
47. Shafik A. Anal submucosal injection: a new route for drug administration. VI. Chronic prostatitis—a new modality treatment with report of eleven cases. *Urology* 1991;37:61.
48. Nickel JC, Sorensen R. Transurethral microwave thermotherapy of nonbacterial prostatitis and prostatodynia: initial experience. *Urology* 1994;44:458.

Antibiotic Therapy in Urology,
edited by S. Grant Mulholland, M.D.,
Lippincott-Raven Publishers, Philadelphia © 1996.

Chapter 6

Antimicrobial Prophylaxis in Genitourinary Surgery

Culley C. Carson III

Division of Urology, University of North Carolina, North Carolina 27599-7235

The routine use of antimicrobial agents for infection prophylaxis in the perioperative period has radically altered surgical practice in the past 30 years. Currently, perioperative antibiotic administration accounts for one of the most frequent indications for use of antibiotics in hospitals. It has been estimated that as many as one-half of all antibiotics prescribed in a hospital setting are used for perioperative prophylaxis (1). Prophylactic perioperative antibiotics have been the subject of many studies, opinions, debates, and controversies. Many randomized trials have demonstrated a reduction in the incidence of postoperative wound infections as a result of perioperative antibiotic administration (2–5). Many other studies, however, have failed to produce data that clearly produce a consensus about prophylactic antibiotics (6–8). While the efficacy of antibiotics in the perioperative period is not firmly established, meticulous surgical techniques—with a minimum of tissue damage, strict adherence to sterile technique, and creation of normal physiologic function without the presence of foreign bodies such as sutures or tubes—remain the cornerstone of prevention of surgical infections.

The classification of surgical wounds as suggested by the American College of Surgeons places most genitourinary surgery in the "clean-contaminated" category if urine remains sterile (9). With infected urine, the procedure falls into the "contaminated" or "infected" class. The use of prophylactic antibiotics for wounds in the clean-contaminated category is controversial (10). Perioperative antibiotics are antimicrobial agents administered in the perioperative period to prevent infections in the postoperative period. In cases of established infection or contamination, such as urosepsis, the term prophylaxis is not appropriate in describing antibiotic treatment; antibiotics in this situation are administered as specific infection treatment rather than as a preventive measure. Thus, administration of antibiotics before prostatectomy, whether transurethral or open, in a patient with established urinary tract infection should be considered as antibiotic treatment, not as perioperative prophylactic antibiotic administration (11).

The potential side effects of antibiotics must be considered prior to their administration in a prophylactic regimen. Allergic reactions, superinfections with resistant bacteria and fungi, and potential bacterial sensitivity variations within the hospital community must be considered before using antibiotics in uninfected patients. If in the opinion of the surgeon these potential risks do not outweigh the benefits, the use of prophylactic antibiotics must be considered inappropriate. In the implantation of foreign bodies, such as penile prostheses or grafts, in potentially contaminated fields, as in cases of trauma and surgery involving the large or small bowel, the benefits of prophylactic antibiotics far outweigh these risks (12).

The costs of antibiotic prophylaxis in hospitalization are considerable. As much as one-quarter of hospital cephalosporin use may be accounted for by perioperative administration (13). Many of the costs associated with prophylactic antibiotic use can be limited by adhering to basic rules of perioperative antibiotic administration (14). Those rules include administering specific antibiotics targeted at organisms suspected to be postoperative infectious agents, limiting the administration of perioperative antibiotics to the immediate perioperative period, and adherence to meticulous surgical technique.

ANTIBIOTIC AGENTS FOR PROPHYLAXIS

Microbiology of Prophylactic Antibiotics Administration

Antimicrobial sensitivities must be considered prior to the administration of any prophylactic perioperative antibiotic agent. Because in a clean-contaminated surgical procedure culture data are unavailable, the most likely infecting agent to cause colonization in each case must be considered on a practical basis. Statistical data from the clinical microbiology laboratory at each hospital are available for defined susceptibilities of bacteria in that institution to specific antimicrobial agents. The bacteria against which prophylactic antibiotics are to be used must be predicted prior to antibiotic administration. In the urologic patient who is undergoing prostatic surgery, wounds are most frequently contaminated with gram-positive organisms, such as *Staphylococcus aureus* and *S. epidermidis*, or gram-negative organisms, such as *Escherichia coli*. Since staphylococci are usually indigenous to the patient's abdominal skin and bowel flora and are not of hospital origin, most of these bacteria are sensitive to multiple antibiotics and usually present a problem only with open prostatic surgery;

these organisms rarely cause postoperative infections after transurethral surgical procedures (15). More than 90% of these infecting bacteria are sensitive to common antibiotics, such as first-generation cephalosporins, tetracyclines, erythromycin, nitrofurantoin, sulfonamides, and fluoroquinolones. Because antimicrobial sensitivities vary from hospital to hospital, knowledge of bacterial sensitivity patterns at each hospital not only facilitates the treatment of bacterial infection but also guides the physician in the selection of an appropriate antibiotic for perioperative prophylaxis in patients who have been hospitalized for prolonged periods prior to their surgery. Surgical procedures that involve significant risk of contamination or infection with gram-negative pathogens should be covered with a different type of antibiotic regimen. These involve entry into the gastrointestinal tract, as in radical cystoprostatectomy, bladder augmentation, or urinary diversion procedures. If gastrointestinal tract entry is predicted prior to surgical procedure, proper preoperative mechanical and antibiotic bowel preparation must be carried out to eliminate colonization with gram-negative organisms such as *E. coli*.

Regardless of the operative procedure planned, however, the appropriate use of prophylactic antibiotics depends largely on the knowledge of the most probable offending organism and its antimicrobial sensitivities at the hospital involved. This knowledge enables the surgeon to decide if prophylactic antibiotic therapy is necessary and, if so, which antibiotic agent will be most effective.

Timing of Administration

Perioperative antibiotics are effective only if administered on an appropriate schedule. In vitro studies performed within the past decades have demonstrated a substantial reduction in the incidence of wound infections when antibiotics are administered prior to surgery. Effective antibiotic levels must be present in the tissue being operated on or the skin to be incised at the time of bacterial contamination for antibiotic prophylaxis to be beneficial (1,2). Therefore, antibiotic agents are most effective when administered 1 to 2 hours before surgery. Antibiotics begun intraoperatively or postoperatively are much less effective in preventing wound infection than those administered prior to the contaminating event. Classen et al. (1) have demonstrated that prophylactic antibiotics are most effective if administered during the 2-hour period prior to the surgical incision. In their study, infection rates increased substantially if antibiotics were begun more than 2 hours preoperatively or in the postoperative period. Their study clearly demonstrates that prophylaxis administration after incision is associated with progressively increased wound infection rates as antibiotic administration is delayed. They also suggest that antibiotics administered more than 2 hours preoperatively undergo an "antibiotic washout," increasing the incidence of wound infection in these patients. Cephalosporin antibiotics administered in their study exhibit half-lives ranging from 40 to 110 minutes. Thus, it is apparent that the surgical wound is at risk for contamination and the initiation of infection is principally during the time between incision and final skin closure. Administration of antibiotics after this time is unlikely to reduce wound infections. Shapiro (16) has suggested that short-acting antibiotics administered in surgery should be repeated during prolonged surgical procedures since an increase in operative time seems to correlate with decreased efficiency of preoperative antibiotics. Burke (2) used an animal model to study optimal time for local tissue response to bacterial contamination. These pioneering investigations initiated a more effective understanding of the opportunities for invention during surgical procedures. These investigators demonstrated that the severity of an infection in laboratory animals was determined within 4 hours of bacterial contamination. After this time, manipulation of host defense mechanisms and administration of antibiotics have little effect on the subsequent infection. Polk and Lopez-Mayor (17) supported these principles in studies of clinical surgery. Stone and associates (3) compared the incidence of postoperative infection in groups of patients treated with antibiotic agents 8 to 12 hours prior to the operation with that in patients receiving cefazolin 1 hour preoperatively. Although tissue antibiotic levels were consistently higher in those patients given cefazolin 8 to 12 hours prior to surgery, the incidence of infection postoperatively was equivalent in both groups. Administration of antibiotics within 2 hours of surgery allows sufficient time for peak serum and tissue levels to be achieved. This principle is especially valid for antibiotics that penetrate tissues rapidly, such as cephalosphorins. More time may be necessary for other agents, such as aminoglycosides, to penetrate tissues sufficiently to provide adequate prophylaxis. Elimination of preoperative antibiotics and a short interval between antibiotic administration and surgery has the added advantage of decreasing the emergence of multiple-drug-resistant bacteria (18,19).

Antibiotics should be discontinued after the threat of bacterial colonization has passed, usually within 36 hours of surgery. Continuation of antibiotics beyond that time increases the risk of drug toxicity and may mask an occult resistant infection (20). The use of a total of two to four doses of perioperative antibiotics beginning in the immediate preoperative period is ideal prophylactic antibiotic treatment for most surgical procedures. Stone et al. (3) have found no advantage to extending the duration of prophylactic antibiotic coverage beyond the day of surgery. If one compares single-dose preoperative antibiotic prophylaxis in gastrointestinal surgery with longer-term antibiotics, the single-dose preoperative regimen is consistently as effective as the multiple-dose prophylaxis. More prolonged prophylactic antibiotic use may be indicated, however, if an occult infection is suspected.

In addition to the surgical procedure, anesthetic agents are known to alter normal physiology and diminish normal host resistance to infection and bacterial contamination (2,4,18). Because the time of bacterial entry into the patient's wound is after the incision, prevention of infection depends on host resistance to active bacterial contamination during this decisive period. The antibiotic should be present at the time of initial incision or cystoscopic prostate evaluation. However, once the surgical procedure is concluded and the patient has returned to normal physiologic responses to infectious agents, the administration of antibiotic agents can only be expected to be harmful. A number of risk factors to the host can be identified. These include coexisting infection at a site remote to the surgical procedure, obesity, diabetes mellitus, and prolonged preoperative hospitalization. The use of immunosuppressive medications such as cyclosporin in transplantation surgery and immunosuppression from HIV infection and AIDS also increases the incidence of perioperative infections. Colonization with organisms such as *S. aureus* in the upper respiratory tract has been also associated with an increase in remote surgical wound infection (21, 22). In patients with these increased risk factors or immunosuppression, careful attention to surgical technique and a carefully designed perioperative antibiotic regimen must be used to diminish the chances of postoperative infections.

PROPHYLACTIC ANTIBIOTICS IN UROLOGIC SURGERY

Over the past 30 years, many studies have been performed to evaluate the place of antibiotic prophylaxis in urologic surgery (4,23). A review of well-designed trials of antibiotic prophylaxis produced little evidence that clearly supported the use of prophylactic antibiotics in urologic surgery (6). Local custom and peer pressure commonly dictate the use of prophylactic antibiotic; in this regard, customs rather that scientific evidence continue to fuel the controversy over the prophylactic use of antibiotics during surgical procedures.

Transurethral Procedures

The lower urinary tract of patients with no significant urologic disease are usually sterile but may be colonized by bacteria of minimal pathogenicity. If simple transurethral instrumentation is performed without adequate instrument sterilization or prior antiseptic skin preparation, urinary tract colonization and subsequent urinary tract infection may ensue. The prevention of bacterial colonization of the urinary tract after simple office cystoscopy for the examination of the urinary tract is preferable to treatment of an active post~instrumentation infection. Even if the urine is sterile, urethral orifices, vaginal surfaces, and urethral channels may contain numerous bacteria (4). These bacteria frequently include *S. epidermidis*, *S. saprophyticus*, diphtheroids, and streptococci. Lactobacilli are usually present on genital surfaces in most healthy women. Appropriate topical antiseptic preparation, therefore, is the best way to prevent post-instrumentation sepsis. Transient bacteremia frequently occurs in patients with bacteriuria or frank urinary tract infection who have undergone genitourinary manipulation. In some of these cases, the bacteremia may result in sepsis or septic shock. This potentially serious complication of urinary instrumentation is most common in male patients who have a urinary tract infection or large postvoid residual urine volumes and inadequate voiding function as a result of obstructive uropathy caused by bacterial prostatitis or benign prostatic hypertrophy. Elective cystourethroscopy, urethral dilation, and other urologic instrumentation should be delayed when bacteriuria is documented. These patients should receive a course of appropriate antimicrobial therapy and have documented sterile urine cultures prior to instrumentation. Thus, a routine cystoscopy in a man with a urinary tract infection is contraindicated. Patients in whom emergent transurethral instrumentation is carried out in the presence of bacteriuria should be protected against bacteremia by appropriate pre-instrumentation prophylactic antibiotics. Coverage of gram-negative organisms such as *E. coli* must be considered in these patients. The use of aminoglycoside, β-lactam, or fluoroquinolone antibiotics is most effective therapy under these circumstances (24). Antibiotics should be continued after the procedure until the urine is sterile. Strictly speaking, this indication for perioperative antibiotics should not be considered prophylactic.

Transurethral instrumentation in more complex situations, such as ureteroscopy, stone manipulation, and endosurgery, presents a more challenging situation. In many of these patients, infection stones are present in the upper urinary tract and seed the urinary tract with bacteria. Fourcade et al. (25) reported their experience in a multicenter, placebo-controlled, double-blinded trial of patients undergoing complex upper urinary procedures for the manipulation and removal of renal calculi. Their study utilized a long-acting cephalosporin antibiotic, cefotaxime, administered as a single 1-g intravenous dose at anesthesia induction. These investigators reported an early postoperative infection rate of 25% in the placebo group, compared with 8.3% in the cefotaxime-treated group. This placebo-controlled study clearly demonstrate the advantages of antibiotic prophylaxis in complex upper urinary tract surgical procedures.

Indwelling Catheters

Antimicrobial therapy in patients with indwelling Foley catheters is seldom necessary. Short-term urethral catheterization with closed-system drainage rarely leads to urinary tract infection (UTI). Catheter-associated UTI should be prevented rather than treated. The closed system of urinary drainage with indwelling urethral catheterization is well established as the most effective prevention of catheter-associated infections. Specific recommendations for appropriate catheter care have been widely published (15,23). All patients should undergo urinalysis and culture after catheter removal. Patients with bacteriuria after catheter removal must be treated with antibiotics as indicated by the antimicrobial sensitivities. Follow-up cultures should then be obtained 1 week after termination of antibiotic treatment. Routine antibiotic coverage of indwelling urethral catheters should not be encouraged because antimicrobial therapy rarely prevents urinary bacterial colonization and only selects resistant organisms in the urine. Likewise, irrigation of catheters with antibiotic or acetic acid solutions compromises the strict principles of the closed-system drainage technique. Such a procedural compromise, although it maintains a sterile urine for a short period of time, ultimately leads to catheter contamination, frequently with multiple-drug-resistant organisms. Therefore, in the absence of fever or acute urinary symptoms associated with UTI, antimicrobial therapy is not required.

Prostatectomy

Prostatectomy, whether transurethral or open, simple or radical, is one of the most common operative procedures performed by urologic surgeons. Because many of the prostates removed show infection in specimen cultures, postoperative infection with these surgical procedures is a significant risk (Table 1).

Recurrent urinary tract infection occurs frequently in men with enlarged prostates, bladder outlet obstruction, and significant postvoid residual urine volumes prior to undergoing transurethral or simple prostatectomy. The most common cause of recurrent urinary tract infection in men is chronic bacterial prostatitis. As many as 60% of resected prostates show significant bacteria on cultures of urine of resected prostate tissue (26). Furthermore, patients with significant bladder outlet obstruction who were catheterized preoperatively or had large residual urines frequently have infected or colonized urine at the time of surgery. Postoperatively, an open healing prostate capsule is left exposed without closure of the surgical incision. This open surface may produce not only urinary infection but also postoperative bacteremia.

TABLE 1. *Perioperative antibiotics for TURP*

- Sterile urine (optional)
  - Parenteral antibiotics: 1–2 hours before surgery
    - First-generation cephalosporin
    - Gentamicin, tobramycin, amikacin
  - Postoperatively 2–4 doses of parenteral antibiotic
- Bacteriuria with prostatic obstruction
  - Parenteral antibiotics: evening before and on call
    - Gentamicin
    - Cephalosporin
  - Postoperatively fluoroquinolone; continue parenteral antibiotic throughout hospitalization
- At discharge
  - 5–10 days' oral antibiotic
    - Trimethoprim/sulfamethoxazole
    - Tetracycline
    - Cephalosporin
    - Fluoroquinolone
  - If *Pseudomonas* preoperatively:
    - Fluoroquinolone
    - Carbenicillin

Numerous studies have compared prophylactic antibiotic treatment regimens with placebo treatment in patients undergoing prostate surgery (4,24,27). Many of these studies, however, lack proper controls, patient selection, or an adequate study design to draw strong conclusions (6). Matthew et al. (28), in a prospective randomized study of 100 patients, demonstrated a significantly greater incidence of post-TURP bacteriuria in patients receiving no antibiotics than in patients receiving nitrofurantoin 6 hours preoperatively and 100 mg three times daily for 10 days postoperatively. Because nitrofurantoin's activity is primarily limited to the urinary tract, conclusions about the results of prophylaxis for bacteremia cannot be drawn from this study. Ramsey and Sheth (4) investigated the effects of perioperative gentamicin administration with a control group of patients. Their study demonstrated a significant increase in postoperative bacteriuria in patients who were not treated with perioperative antibiotics. Comparison of their three different administration schedules failed to reveal a statistically significant difference between patients who received a single dose of gentamicin 2 hours prior to surgery, those who received antibiotics 12 hours prior to surgery, and those who received a 5-day postoperative course of gentamicin following an initial preoperative dose. Cox (29) compared intravenous ciprofloxacin and intravenous cefotaxime as antimicrobial prophylaxis in elderly men undergoing transurethral prostatic resection procedures. He reported an equivalent postoperative infection rate between the two groups of patients but decreased distant infection rates during the post-hospital recovery time for those patients treated initially with intravenous ciprofloxacin. Grabe (11) demonstrated a 3% incidence of bacteriuria in patients treated with perioperative ciprofloxacin, compared with a 19% incidence of postoperative bacteriuria in a control group. The difference in these numbers was significantly increased when patients with preoperative bacteriuria were studied: there was a 9% postoperative infection rate in patients with long-term perioperative antibiotic coverage, compared with a 92% incidence of postoperative bacteriuria in the control patients. A similar disparity in postoperative bacteriuria was found by Grabe (11) in a study using cefotaxime. The significance of increased bacteriuria was even more dramatic when those patients who had preoperative catheter drainage prior to transurethral resection of the prostate were evaluated. Interestingly, however, no statistically significant difference was found between groups when observing postoperative fever. Similar data were obtained by Prokocimer et al. using a double-blinded, randomized trial with cefotaxime (30). Several other studies using combinations of antibiotics have reported similar results (5,24). However, many uncontrolled or poorly controlled studies reported no significance between antibiotic-treated and placebo groups.

Landes et al. (26) investigated more than 400 patients who underwent TURP and were evaluated with urine and prostate tissue cultures. Their data clearly showed that the incidence of postoperative bacteriuria and morbidity caused by infection was lowest in patients whose urine was sterile prior to surgery. Of the infected patients, only 12% developed postoperative bacteriuria. Patients who had preoperative bacteriuria and whose urine was sterilized with appropriate antimicrobials also had minimal postoperative bacteriuria. The greatest morbidity occurred in a group of 81 patients who had bacteriuria preoperatively with infected prostate tissue specimens but received no preoperative medication. Of this group, 23% developed postoperative bacteriuria. These patients had a significantly longer hospital stay and higher urinary and systemic infection rates. The patients with the highest morbidity were those in whom the culture of the prostate chips revealed significant prostate tissue infection.

Madsen et al. (31) also investigated the effects of perioperative prophylactic antibiotics in transurethral prostatectomy. They compared a group of patients who received cefoxitin 1 to 2 hours prior to TURP and continued treatment as long as they had an indwelling catheter with a control group of patients treated only with placebo. Their results indicate infection at 3 days in 26.4% of placebo-treated patients, compared with only 3.9% in those patients treated with antibiotics. At 7 days the difference continued; 42% of placebo-treated patients demonstrated infection, whereas only 6.5% of cefoxitin-treated patients had bacteriuria.

The authors were unable to correlate post-TURP infection with other infection risk factors, such as age, general patient condition, diagnosis, operating time, preoperative instrumentation, weight of resected tissue, or intraoperative blood loss. Similarly, there was no difference in the incidence or degree of postoperative fever between the two groups of patients.

Appropriate systemic antibiotic therapy should be given to patients prior to prostatic surgery, especially if preoperative bacteriuria is present (32). This antibiotic treatment should be based on carefully collected urine specimens and their antimicrobial sensitivities. The rational choice of an antimicrobial agent in these situations must consider the pharmacokinetic properties of the antibiotic to be used. Antibiotics that are effective only in the urinary tract, without tissue penetration or systemic effectiveness, are unsuitable perioperatively for transurethral resection of the prostate. Nitrofurantoin, methenamine mandelate, and similar agents cannot be expected to eradicate prostatic tissue infections.

In patients with sterile preoperative urine and no preoperative catheterization or large residual urines, antimicrobial prophylaxis may be unnecessary. Postoperative urine culture should be obtained following the removal of the indwelling Foley catheter in these cases, however, to determine if antibiotics should be begun prior to hospital discharge.

The origin of bacteriuria after TURP remains an enigma. By studying and culturing prostate chips taken from transurethral resections, several studies have suggested that the prostate tissue itself is frequently contaminated at the time of surgery (23,26). More likely, however, infecting bacteria enter the bladder and the healing prostatic tissue transurethrally while the Foley catheter is in place (33). With postoperative infection rates above 25% in many studies of control patients without antibiotic treatment, it would seem prudent to conclude that prophylactic antibiotics should be used in TURP. The major controversy, however, concerns the duration of prophylaxis. In our present era of cost consciousness and with concern over development of resistant bacteria in the hospital setting, it would seem that the shortest effective period of prophylaxis should be used. To this end, the study by Ramsey and Sheth (4) and by Grabe (11) demonstrated no significant difference between groups treated only preoperatively and those treated throughout hospitalization. Thus, only perioperative antibiotics should be used, followed by a urine culture after removal of the Foley catheter as a guide to further postoperative antibiotic treatment.

Other Genitourinary Surgery

Many of the surgical procedures unique to urology require special consideration for antibiotic use. Upper urinary tract endoscopic procedures may be associated with significant urinary tract infection. As many as 20% of urinary calculi may be associated with infection and urea-splitting uropathogenic organisms. In these situations, temporary sterilization of the urinary tract with antibiotics to allow safe endourologic intervention is critical. It must be considered, however, that cessation of therapy results in rapid return of bacteria (34). Percutaneous and ureteroscopic procedures to remove calculi and perform endosurgical techniques have changed the specialty of urology and the use of prophylactic antibiotics. Stone fragmentation, whether endourologic or extracorporeal, may liberate viable bacteria previously contained within the stone, increasing the risk for bacteremia (35). While these stones cannot be sterilized preoperatively, perioperative antibiotics usually decrease the chances of postoperative septic complications. It has been reported that percutaneous stone surgery is associated with temperature elevation in approximately 10% of cases (35,36). Approximately 35% of cases may have associated urinary tract infection (25). Uncontrolled studies have demonstrated a reduction in this postoperative infection rate to less than 3% (37). Fourcade et al. (25), in a multicenter, placebo-controlled, double-blinded study, reported a postoperative bacteriuria incidence of 25% in a placebo group, compared with only 8.5% in a perioperative cefotaxime-treated group. Postoperative fever was reduced from 20% in the placebo group to less than 15% in the antibiotic-treated patients. Cefotaxime, a long-acting cephalosporin, was administered in a single 1-g intravenous dose at the induction of anesthesia in their patients.

No well-controlled or objective studies have been carried out to investigate the role of antibiotic prophylaxis in extracorporeal shock-wave lithotripsy (ESWL). Although fever follows ESWL in 15–25% of patients, Westh et al. in a study of 55 ESWL patients confirmed the small incidence of post-ESWL bacteremia (38,39). It would seem appropriate, however, that patients having a positive urine culture or a suspected of having infection stones be treated prior to surgery as well as perioperatively with antibiotics aimed at urea-splitting organisms, especially *Proteus* (40,41). Charton et al. (40) have reviewed 400 patients treated with ESWL for renal and ureteral stones. Of 278 patients with no history of previous bacteriuria or instrumentation, 95.2% had neither fever nor bacteriuria post-ESWL, suggesting that perioperative antibiotics are not necessary in this group. This opinion was confirmed by Petterson and Tiseleus (41). In their 89 patients with preoperative urinary tract infection treated with at least 12 hours of sensitivity-specific antibiotics and continued for 10 or more days after treatment, 78.7% did not develop fever or bacteriuria. Three patients with transient obstruction and two without obstruction with preoperative bacteriuria developed septic shock despite appropriate antibiotics. The authors concluded that a 5-day pretreatment antibiotic program would most effectively eliminate post-treatment infection and sepsis. Since ESWL produces significant renal microtrauma (36) and since bacteriuria and bacteremia can be expected after liberating bacteria from infection stones, perioperative antibiotics must be administered in these patients with possible infection stones. ESWL energy application cannot be expected to be bactericidal (42). Most appropriate antibiotic coverage for these suspected infection stones would be a first-generation cephalosporin or ampicillin in addition to an aminoglycoside administered 1 to 2 hours before lithotripsy and continued for 24 hours postoperatively or until the patient is afebrile for at least 24 hours. If significant *steinstrasse* is encountered, antibiotics must be continued until free urine flow has been restored. Since *Proteus* is not initially retrieved from all patients with suspected infection stones, broad-spectrum antibiotic coverage must be provided since bacteria in deep portions of the stone may represent *Pseudomonas* or other difficult-to-treat gram-negative pathogens. In those patients with suspected or proven infection stones, our usual protocol requires preoperative administration of oral antibiotics for 7 to 10 days prior to ESWL. Agents such as trimethoprim/sulfamethoxazole, cephalosporin, ampicillin, carbenicillin, or a fluoroquinolone may be helpful in these patients. In patients at high risk for endocarditis or with risk factors such as obesity, diabetes mellitus, azotemia, or implanted prostheses, antibiotic prophylaxis should be administered routinely (42,43).

In patients in whom long-term indwelling ureteral stenting is necessary following endosurgery or stone manipulation, prophylactic antibiotics may be required along with suppressive antibiotics in the post-stent placement period (43,44). Since a foreign body is to be placed in the urinary tract, maintaining a sterile urine may not be possible, and in patients who are asymptomatic with adequate urine drainage, broad-spectrum antibiotics may serve only to select resistant organisms. Colonization of the urine, however, can be expected to increase the rate of stent encrustation and increase the potential for stent obstruction (45). It is our practice for short-term indwelling ureteral stent placement to administer suppressive antibiotics while the stent is in place. In these cases, trimethoprim/sulfamethoxazole or cephalosporin may be the most appropriate antibiotic. During stent replacement procedures, preoperative antibiotics such as an aminoglycoside and cephalosporin are most effective.

Urologic Prosthetic Surgery

Perioperative antibiotic administration is especially advantageous with urologic prosthetic surgery. Infections in these situations can be disastrous to the outcome of the procedure and must be vigorously prevented. While placebo-controlled studies in these situations are impossible, one can draw some conclusions from published reports of prosthetic infections. In early reports of penile prosthesis surgery, Small (46) reported a decrease in postoperative infections from more than 15% to approximately 1% when perioperative antibiotics were employed. With the routine use of perioperative infections, infections associated with penile prostheses and artificial urinary sphincters can be expected to occur in approximately 2% of patients (47). The most common organisms associated with these prosthesis infections include gram-positive cocci, such as *S. epidermidis* and *S. aureus*, and gram-negative organisms, such as *E. coli*, *Proteus*, and *Pseudomonas*. Since a foreign body is employed in these procedures, colonizing bacteria may produce a biofilm that surrounds the prosthetic material and harbors bacteria but is impenetrable to circulating antibiotics and host defense mechanisms. Preoperatively, remote infection, including bacteriuria, must be eliminated to decrease the incidence of post-prosthetic implantation infections. Similarly, once the prosthetic device has been implanted, remote infections have been reported, and antibiotics should be suggested for patients undergoing lower gastrointestinal tract manipulation, complex dental procedures, and other operations likely to result in bacteremia (48).

In these prosthetic procedures, first-generation cephalosporins, penicillinase-resistant semisynthetic penicillins, and ampicillin are effective prophylactic antibiotic agents. If a patient has a penicillin allergy, a combination of vancomycin and an aminoglycoside is an effective alternative (47). Our usual perioperative antibiotic protocol includes a first generation-cephalosporin and an aminoglycoside administered 1 to 2 hours prior to surgery followed by 48 hours of intravenous antibiotic prophylaxis using this same combination. In patients who are allergic to β-lactam antibiotics, vancomycin is substituted for the cephalosporin agent.

Suppressive Antibiotics for Prostate Biopsy

Currently, biopsies of the prostate are performed by aspiration through a needle placed transrectally or transperineally with digital or ultrasonographic localization. Because of bacterial colonization of skin and rectal mucosa, infection can easily follow these procedures. The administration of prophylactic antibiotics prior to prostatic biopsy is currently the standard practice in most hospitals (Table 2). Transperineal biopsies tend to be associated with fewer infections than transrectal biopsies because of the cleaner area through which the needle passes. Few studies are available that examine the effects of prophylactic antibiotics with perineal biopsy. Russo et al. (49) reported a retrospective study of 162 patients who had undergone transperineal prostate biopsy. Of these patients, 4.3% had a febrile episode after biopsy but only 2% had culture-proven urinary tract infection. Only one of these patients had a symptomatic urinary tract infection. Their conclusion was that in patients with sterile

TABLE 2. *Preparation for prostate biopsy*

Transrectal	
	Cleansing enema 2–4 hours before biopsy
Transrectal and transperineal perioperative antibiotics	
	Gentamicin 80 mg 1–2 h before biopsy
	Tetracycline 1 g 1–2 h before biopsy and 500 mg qid for 24 h after biopsy
	Ciprofloxicin 500 mg 1–2 h before biopsy and 500 mg bid for 24 h after biopsy

urine, transperineal needle biopsy should be considered a clean procedure requiring only a standard sterile technique and preoperative preparation of the area traversed by the needle and that perioperative antibiotics are necessary.

Several studies are available that examine the effects of prophylactic antimicrobial agents in transrectal needle biopsy. Transrectal needle biopsies are more commonly associated with urinary tract infectin, fever, and bacteremia than transperineal needle biopsies. Occasionally, patients with transrectal needle biopsies experience postbiopsy epididymitis, upper urinary tract infections, prostate abscesses, prostate tissue infections, and symptoms of urosepsis. Ruebush and associates (50) examined the effects of perioperative antibiotics using trimiethoprim/sulfamethoxazole compared with a placebo. Their study demonstrated no significant difference in the incidence of transient bacteremia or fever in the two groups. Transient bacteremia was identified in 70% of their population. Prophylactic antibiotics administered prior to transrectal needle biopsy, however, significantly reduced the incidence of bacteriuria in comparison with placebo. In a group of 16,044 patients undergoing transrectal needle biopsies at the Mayo Clinic, 7 patients had postbiopsy septicemia within 24 hours of the procedure (51). All patients in the Mayo Clinic series recovered satisfactorily with hospitalization and postbiopsy parenteral antibiotic treatment.

Crawford and associates (23) compared the effects of carbenicillin, indanyl sodium, and a placebo in the perioperative period and reported significantly fewer episodes of postoperative bacteriuria and fever in 63 antibiotic-treated patients. Although transient bacteremia was identified in similar numbers in both groups, gram-negative sepsis occurred in three placebo patients compared with only one patient in the antibiotic treatment group. This case of sepsis was caused by *Klebsiella* and was resistant to carbenicillin.

As a result of these studies and the fact that penetration of the gastrointestinal tract classifies a surgical procedure as contaminated, prophylactic, broad-spectrum, perioperative antibiotics should be administered to patients undergoing transrectal needle biopsy of the prostate. In the two series in which patients sustained sepsis, five patients grew *E.*

coli and three patients grew *Klebsiella* (50,52). As a result, it is imperative that antibiotic coverage be targeted towards these organisms and other gram-negative organisms prior to prostate biopsy (52).

Selection of Perioperative Antibiotic Agents

In those cases in which perioperative antibiotic treatment is necessary for prophylaxis, an appropriate agent must be chosen for the prevention of the suspected infection (Table 3). Agents that are strictly effective within the urinary tract and do not achieve reasonable serum and tissue levels are inappropriate for perioperative antibiotic programs. Such agents as methenamine and nitrofurantoin are active only in the urinary tract and are generally inappropriate for perioperative antibiotic use. Cephalosporins may be effective against penicillinase-producing staphylococci and many community-acquired *E. coli* and *Klebsiella*. First-generation cephalosporins, while less expensive, are not effective against *Proteus*, *Pseudomonas*, resistant *E. coli*, and many enterococci. Third-generation cephalosporins cover the spectrum of bacteria that may be responsible for post-prostatectomy infections. These agents, however, are extremely expensive and may be restricted at many hospitals. Agents such as cefotaxime, cefoperazone, ceftriaxone, and cefonicid are examples of these third-generation cephalosporins that may be effective as prophylactic agents but are far too costly for routine use. For urologic surgery involving the colon or rectum, a second- or third-generation cephalosporin such as cefoxitin or cefotetan is a more appropriate choice than a first-generation cephalosporin since these are more active against gastrointestinal anaerobes such as *Bacteroides fragilis*. Third-generation cephalosporin agents, in addition to their expense, have poor activity against staphylococci, and their spectrum of ac-

TABLE 3. *Perioperative antibiotic choices*

Agent[a]	Dose
Cefazolin	1 g IM on call + q6h × 4 doses
Cefotaxime	1 g IM on call + q6h. × 4 doses
Cefoperazone	2 g IM on call + 12 hours
Ceftriaxone	1 g IM on call
Cefonicid	1 g IM on call
Gentamicin	1.5 mg/kg on call + q8h × 3 doses
Tobramycin	1.5 mg/kg on call + q8h × 3 doses
Amikacin	1.5 mg/kg on call + q8h × 3 doses
Ofloxicin	400 mg IV on call + q12h × 2 doses
Ciprofloxicin	400 mg IV on call + q12h × 2 doses

[a]All prophylactic antibiotics must be given 1–2 h prior to surgery and continued for up to 72 h after surgery.

tion against gram-negative bacilli is too broad for commonly encountered bacteria in elective surgery. Their widespread use can be expected to promote the emergence of multiple-antibiotic-resistant organisms.

Aminoglycosides such as gentamycin, tobramycin, amikacin, netilmicin, and fosfomycin are potent broad-spectrum antibiotics that are effective against many gram-negative organisms causing perioperative urologic infections. These organisms include *E. coli*, *Pseudonomas*, *Klebsiella*, *Serratia*, and *Proteus*. Aminoglycosides, however, are less effective against gram-positive organisms such as staphylococci and enterococci. Their major drawback is the possibility of nephrotoxicity and ototoxicity and the necessity to administer them parenterally. Because perioperative antibiotics are limited to a preoperative dose and a 42- to 72-hour administration postoperatively, parenteral agents are usually the most effective choice. The combination of these aminoglycosides with a first-generation cephalosporin, ampicillin, or other β-lactam antibiotic provide excellent coverage at a reasonable cost.

Fluoroquinolones are a new class of antibiotic agent that may be effective as perioperative antibacterial treatment for selected patients who are able to receive oral agents prior to surgery (53). These antibacterial agents are most effective when gram-negative organisms are suspected. Their excellent penetration of prostate tissue also makes them quite helpful in patients undergoing prostate surgery who have prostate tissue infections or a history of prostatitis. The excellent penetration of urine and prostate fluid by currently available agents such as ciprofloxicin, norfloxicin, and ofloxicin makes these agents extremely helpful for outpatient prostate biopsies. The current availability of ciprofloxicin and ofloxicin as an intravenous preparation allow their use as a perioperative antibiotic for stone surgery and other surgical procedures requiring a broader-spectrum antibiotic coverage, especially in patients with renal compromise.

Antibiotic Prophylaxis for Bacterial Endocarditis

Antibacterial prophylaxis prior to urologic surgical procedures and diagnostic manipulations to prevent bacterial endocarditis in patients with valvular heart disease, cardiac abnormalities, and previous cardiac surgery has been recommended for many years (54) (Table 4). Recently, data have appeared that support the use of prophylactic antibiotics in patients with noncardiac prostheses who are undergoing genitourinary manipulations (18,48). However, no data are available from well-controlled clinical studies to support the use of these agents in the prevention of transient bacteremia. Most clinicians, however, use appropriate perioperative antibacterial agents because infection in these patients can prove disastrous.

TABLE 4. *Antibiotic prophylaxis for bacterial endocarditis*

Standard regimen	
Ampicillin, amoxicillin, gentamicin	IV or IM ampicillin 2.0 g plus gentamicin 1.5 mg/kg (80 mg maximum) 30–60 min before surgery. Repeat parenteral dose after 8 h or 1.5 g ampicillin after 8 h.
Regimen for β-lactam-allergic patient	
Vancomycin and gentamicin	IV vancomycin 1 g over 1 h plus IV or IM gentamicin 1.5 mg/kg (80 mg maximum) 60 min before procedure. Repeat once 8 h later.
Regimen for low-risk patient	
Amoxicillin	3.0 g po 60 min before procedure, 1.5 g po 6 h later.

The indications for prophylaxis include valvular heart disease, prosthetic heart valves, congenital cardiac malformations, total joint replacements, penile prostheses, and other synthetic prosthetic materials. Animal studies suggest regimens administered parenterally are most effective in the prevention of bacteremia in these high-risk patients. Parenteral regimens are especially effective in patients with prosthetic heart valves and in those taking long-term oral penicillin as rheumatic fever prophylaxis. The American Heart Association does not recommend antibiotic prophylaxis for routine urethral catheterization in the absence of infection but does recommend endocarditis prophylaxis in high-risk patients undergoing cystoscopy, urethral dilation, urinary tract surgery, or incision and drainage of infected tissue (18,54).

The standard recommended regimen for patients undergoing genitourinary procedures includes the intravenous or intramuscular administration of 2 g of ampicillin plus 1.5 mg/kg of gentamicin not to exceed 80 mg 30 minutes before the procedure (54). This initial antibiotic coverage should be followed by 1.5 g of amoxicillin every 6 hours beginning 8 hours after the initial dose. An alternate low-risk patient regimen suggested includes 3 g of amoxicillin orally 1 hour before the procedure and 1.5 g of amoxicillin 6 hours following the initial dose. Patients who are β-lactam-antibiotic-allergic may receive initial intravenous administration of 1 g of vancomycin over 1 hour plus intravenous or intramuscular administration of 1.5 mg/kg of gentamicin not to exceed 80 mg 1 hour prior to the procedure. This should then be repeated 8 hours following the initial dose.

REFERENCES

1. Classen DC, Evans RS, Pestotink SL, et al. The timing of prophylactic administration of antibiotics and the risk of surgical wound infection. *N Eng J Med* 1992;326:281.

2. Burke JF. The effective period of preventative antibiotic action in experimental incisions and dermal lesions. *Surgery* 1961;50:161.
3. Stone HH, Hooper CA, Colby LD, et al. Antibiotic prophylaxis in gastric, biliary and colonic surgery. *Ann Surg* 1976;184:443.
4. Ramsey EW, Sheth NK. Antibiotic prophylaxis in patients undergoing prostatectomy. *Urology* 1983;21:367.
5. Murphy DM, Stassen L, Car R, et al. Bacteremia following prostatectomy and other transurethral operations: influence of timing of antibiotic administration. *J Clin Path* 1984;37:673.
6. Chodak GW, Plant ME. Systemic antibiotics for prophylaxis and urologic surgery: critical review. *J Urol* 1979;121:695.
7. Dellinger EP. Design and evaluation of clinical trials of antimicrobial agents in surgery. *Surg Gynecol Obstet* 1991;172:65.
8. Van Scoy RE, Wilkowske CJ. Prophylactic use of antimicrobial agents in adult patients. *Mayo Clin Proc* 1992;67:288.
9. Altemeier WA, Burke JF, Pruitt BA, et al. *Manual of control of infection in surgical patients.* Philadelphia: JB Lippincott; 1976;141:8.
10. Cluver DH, Horan TC, Gaynes RP. Surgical wound infection rates by wound class, operative procedure, and patient risk index. *Am J Med* 1991;91:152S.
11. Grabe M. Antimicrobial agents in transurethral prostatic resection. *J Urol* 1987;138:245.
12. Galandiuk S, Polk HC, Jagelman DG, et al. Re-emphasis of priorities in surgical antibiotic prophylaxis. *Surg Gynecol Obstet* 1989;169:219.
13. Scalley RD, Irwin AD, Paduska PJ, et al. Surgical antibiotic prophylaxis, patient morbidity and cost reduction: a three year study. *Drug Intel Clin Pharm* 1987;21:648.
14. Scher KS, Bernstein JM, Arenstein GL, et al. Reducing the cost of surgical prophylaxis. *Am Surg* 1990;56:32.
15. Carson CC. Prophylactic antibiotics in urologic surgery. *Weekly Urology Update Series* 1979;26:1.
16. Shapiro M. Perioperative prophylactic use of antibiotics in surgery: principles and practice. *Infect Control* 1982;3:38.
17. Polk HC, Lopez-Mayor JF. Postoperative wound infections: a prospective study of determinant factors in prevention. *Surgery* 1969;66:97.
18. Abramowicz M (ed.). Antimicrobial prophylaxis in surgery. *Med Lett* 1992;34:5.
19. Fry DE. Antibiotics in surgery: an overview. *Am J Surg* 1988;155:11.
20. Neu HC. Clinicopharmakinetics in preventative antimicrobial therapy. *South Med J* 1977;70:14.
21. Kaiser AB. Antimicrobial prophylaxis in surgery. *N Eng J Med* 1986;315:1129.
22. Yu VL, Goetz A, Wagener M, et al. Staphylococcus aureus nasal carriage and infection in patients on hemodialysis: efficacy of antibiotic prophylaxis. *N Eng J Med* 1986;315:91.
23. Crawford ED, Hanes AL, Story MW. Prevention of urinary tract infection and sepsis following transrectal prostate biopsy. *J Urol* 1982;127:449.
24. Larsen EH, Gasser TC, Madsen PO. Antimicrobial prophylaxis in urologic surgery. *Urol Clin North Am* 1986;13:591.
25. Fourcade RO, et al. Antibiotic prophylaxis with cefotaxime in endoscopic extraction of upper urinary tract stones: a randomized study. *J Antimicrob Chemother* 1990;26:77.
26. Landes RR, Medenbach K, Lee RE. Effect of perioperative antibiotic therapy on bacterial prostatitis after transurethral prostatectomy. *Urology* 1986;8:450.
27. Christensen MM, Nielsen KT, Knes J, et al. Brief report: single dose preoperative prophylaxis and transurethral surgery. *Am J Med* 1989;87:258S.
28. Matthew AD, Gonzalez R, Jeffords D, et al. Prevention of bacteriuria after transurethral prostatectomy with nitrofurantoin macrocrystals. *J Urol* 1978;120:442.
29. Cox CE. Comparison of intravenous ciprofloxacin and intravenous cefotaxime for antimicrobial prophylaxis in transurethral surgery. *Am J Med* 1989;87:252S.
30. Prokocimer P, Quazza M, Gilbert CC, et al. Short term prophylactic antibiotics in patients undergoing prostatectomy: report of a double blind randomized trial of two intravenous doses of cefotaxime. *J Urol* 1986;135:60.
31. Madsen PO, Larsen EH, Derflinger T. The role of antimicrobial prophylaxis and urologic surgery. *Urology* 1985;26:35.

32. Hofer DR, Schoeffer AJ. Use of antimicrobials for patients undergoing prostatectomy. *Urol Clin North Am* 1990;17:595.
33. Braehmer B, Madsen PO. Route of prophylaxis of ascending bladder infection in male patients with indwelling catheters. *J Urol* 1972;108:719.
34. Thompson RB, Stamey T. Bacteriology of infected stones. *Urology* 1973;2:627.
35. Tanaka M, Matsumoto T, Kitada S, et al. Endotoxemia in patients who underwent ultrasonic lithotripsy or extracorporeal shock wave lithotripsy. *Eur Urol* 1988;14:173.
36. Charton M, Vallancin G, Veillon B, et al. Urinary tract infection and percutaneous surgery for renal calculi. *J Urol* 1986;135:15.
37. Tauzin-Fin P, Ragnaud JM, Ballanger P, et al. Etude comparitif de la cèphoperazone et du cotrimoxazole dans la chirurgie lithiasique rènale par voie per cutanèe. *Pathologie Biologie* 1986;34:498.
38. Naber KG. Role of antimicrobial prophylaxis in urologic intervention. *Curr Opin Urol* 1992;2:44.
39. Westh H, Knudson F, Hedrengren AM, et al. Extracorporeal shock wave lithotripsy of kidney stones does not induce transient bacteremia. *J Urol* 1990;144:15.
40. Charton M, Vallencien G, Veillon B, et al. Use of antibiotics in conjunction with extracorporeal lithotripsy. *Eur Urol* 1990;17:134.
41. Petterson B, Tiselius HG. Are prophylactic antibiotics necessary during extracorporeal lithotripsy. *Brit J Urol* 1989;63:449.
42. Matlow AG, Goldberg SD. Extracorporeal shock wave lithotripsy and prophylaxis for endocarditis. *Ann Intern Med* 1986;105:966.
43. Saltzman B. Ureteral stents. *Urol Clin North Am* 1988;15:481.
44. Spirnak JP, Resnick MI. Stone formation as a complication of indwelling ureteral stents: report of 5 cases. *J Urol* 1985;134:349.
45. Small MP. Surgical treatment of impotence with Small-Carrion prosthesis. *Urology* 1984;23(Suppl):93.
46. Carson CC. Infections in genitourinary prostheses. *Urol Clin North Am* 1989;16:139.
47. Carson CC, Robertson CN. Late hematogenous infections of penile prostheses. *J Urol* 1988;138:50.
48. Russo P, Packer MG, Fair WR. Prophylactic antibiotics in urologic surgery. *Semin Urol* 1983;1:155.
49. Ruebush TK, McConville JH, Galia FM. A double blind study of trimethoprim-sulfamethoxazole prophylaxis in patients having transrectal biopsy of the prostate. *J Urol* 1979;122:492.
50. Edson RS, van Scoy RE, Leary FJ. Gram negative bacteremia after transrectal needle biopsy of the prostate. *Mayo Clin Proc* 1980;55:49.
51. Melekos MD. Efficacy of prophylactic antimicrobial regimens in preventing infectious complications after transrectal biopsy of the prostate. *Int Urol Nephrol* 1990;22:257.
52. Mandell LA. Role of quinolones in surgical prophylaxis. *Eur J Clin Microbiol Infect Dis* 1991;10:368.
53. Dajani AS, Bisno AL, Chung AJ, et al. Prevention of bacterial endocarditis: recommendations by the American Heart Association. *JAMA* 1990;264:2919.

Antibiotic Therapy in Urology,
edited by S. Grant Mulholland, M.D.,
Lippincott-Raven Publishers, Philadelphia © 1996.

Chapter 7

Diagnosis and Therapy of Clinical and Subclinical Prosthetic Infections

C. Lowell Parsons

Division of Urology, School of Medicine, University of California in San Diego, San Diego, California 92103-8897

ABSTRACT

Both clinically and subclinically infected prostheses are currently the major cause for device failures. These infections may be manifested by the classic overt signs of rubor, dolor, and calor, in which case they are no problem for the clinician to diagnose. On the other hand, subclinically infected implants are frequently not recognized. These infections are manifested by chronic persistent or intermittent pain. When overt or subclinical infection occurs, it can be treated initially with antibiotics that are effective against *Staphylococcus epidermidis*. Overt infection can sometimes be cured or converted to a subclinical infection with medication. If either type of infection is not cured, exchanging the infected device (at the same operation) has a 90% chance of success and precludes the problem with device removal and subsequent problems that occur with attempts to reoperate.

INTRODUCTION

Mechanical dysfunction of urologic prostheses is steadily decreasing as a reason for device failure as compared with infection. Traditionally, one considers prosthetic infections only when manifested by obvious clinical signs, consisting of erythema, pain, collection of white cells, and fever. Frequently, the possibility of infection is not considered until an infection reaches an obvious clinical stage, when the fact is that in most cases the only symptom of bacterial contamination may be chronic pain. Chronic pain is seen with all types of prosthetic material placed in the body, whether it be a breast prosthesis, an orthopedic device, a penile prosthesis, or even nonabsorbable suture material.

In the majority of cases, the primary cause of the pain is infection by *Staphylococcus epidermidis* (1–8).

This review focuses on obvious clinical infections and also on alerting the physician to recognize the existence of "subclinically infected penile prostheses"—those that do not necessarily extrude or have draining abscesses but are associated with chronic, continuous, or intermittent pain. While urology was one of the last specialties to become involved with the implantation of artificial devices, ironically urologists were among the first to recognize that chronic pain associated with devices is usually secondary to infection (9–10). Proving that there was a bacterial cause of the pain was difficult, and most clinicians may accept these conditions as part of having a prosthesis in place, a type of "silicone reaction," or a sqeamish patient overly sensitive to pain. It was our concept that a painful prosthesis was infected at the time of implantation (10). Bacteria so introduced are relatively indolent and produce a subclinical state of infection manifested by chronic pain that may be intermittent in nature. By recognizing this low-grade infection, the surgeon can take measures to prevent or treat it. Such methods will be reviewed.

PATHOGENESIS

Clinically Infected Prostheses

Recognition of the clinically infected prosthetic device is relatively straightforward. The usual signs of fever, pain, and purulent drainage from the wound site make it relatively clear as to what the problem is. Certain clinical settings also increase the likelihood of problems, such as the diabetic individual whose infection rate is substantially increased over that of other patients. The infecting organism is usually *Staphylococcus epidermidis* in penile prosthetic devices, with a scattering of other organisms, particularly gram-negative rods. In the case of other mechanical apparatuses, such as artificial sphincters, when the individual may be incontinent of urine, gram-negative bacteria play a more clinically important role in terms of prosthetic infection. The time of entry of the organisms into the wound and onto prosthetic devices, as in subclinical infection, is at the time of surgery.

Subclinically Infected Prostheses

While urologists recognized early in their use of penile implants that painful prostheses may be infected (10–12), it is not so simple to prove that this is the case. Infections appear to be primarily confined to the surface of the silicone, that is, the bacteria are on the device only with essentially no microorganisms in the adjacent tissue. Nor is the entire surface of the implant necessarily covered by microorganisms. Thus, attempts to culture for *Staphylococcus epidermidis* can be unsuccessful and misleading; culturing the space around the silicone or even swabbing the surface of the device may not yield any viable organisms, since they are enveloped in an invisible biofilm that is firmly adherent to the surface of the silicone (11). The best way to document the presence of infection is to take a piece of the implant and drop it directly into culture medium and incubate for 72 hours. However, when using this culture method, it could be argued that in removing the device the urologist may, during the surgical procedure, incidentally contaminate the prosthesis with skin bacteria, which could account for the positive cultures. To determine whether or not a painful device was truly infected, we cultured both breast and penile prostheses that were being removed either for chronic pain or for mechanical reasons (10).

As can be seen in Table 1, devices that were removed (for mechanical reasons) that were not associated with pain had only a 13% positive culture rate, while devices being removed for pain had a 93% positive culture rate. This is solid evidence supporting the hypothesis that the pain was secondary to chronic low-grade infection. We believe prostheses become contaminated at the time of surgical placement and not subsequently. This contamination is able to "smolder" indefinitely, since *Staphylococcus epidermidis* is not too virulent. The questions of how or whether to treat this "subclinical" infection and to prevent its development are important to answer for the surgeon. If the implant has to be removed because of infection and is not replaced, the scarring and fibrosis that result make it extremely difficult to return at a later time to place a new prosthetic device. Consequently, a method not only to prevent an infection but also to resolve it without removal would be invaluable to the clinician.

Experimental investigations in our laboratory showed that one could disrupt the biofilm of the bacteria by using a substance known to adhere to mucus and thereby interfere with its ability to control permeability. That substance is a quaternary amine, protamine sulfate (13–15). When *Staphylococcus epidermidis* infection was examined both in vitro and in an in vivo silicone infection model in rodents, it was discovered that a

TABLE 1. *Rates of infection (positive culture) of removed prostheses*

Device	Pain, No. (%)	No pain, No. (%)
Penile prostheses	13/14	0/5
Breast prostheses	10/11	4/16
Tissue expanders	3/3	0/10
TOTALS	26/28 (93%)*	4/31 (13%)

*$p < 0.001$, pain vs. no pain.

TABLE 2. *Rates of infection in variously treated groups of rats*

Group[p]	No. evaluable	No. infected	No. sterile	Infection rate, %
Control	12	10	3	77
Vancomycin	24	12	12	50
PS	21	14	7	67
Vancomycin + PS	26	5	21	19

PS, protamine sulfate.
[p] p = 0.05, vancomycin + PS vs. vancomycin; $p < 0.005$, vancomycin + PS vs. PS; $p > 0.5$, vancomycin vs. PS; $p < 0.005$, vancomycin + PS vs. control; $p = 0.5$, control vs. PS; p : 0.2, vancomycin vs. control.

combination of protamine and vancomycin was far more effective at killing the organism or eradicating it from the silicone than either compound alone (16,17). The basic concept was that the bacteria grow on the surface of the device enveloped in their biofilm composed of mucus. One can disrupt the mucus by first exposing it to protamine to destroy its permeability control effect and then add the antibiotic to which the bacteria are sensitive. The results suggested that irrigating a wound with antibiotics has little effect on infected prosthetic devices, but that when an antibiotic is combined with protamine, it is quite successful at reducing the experimentally induced silicone infection in rats (See Table 2).

Based on these experimental observations, we have made several recommendations for both preventing and potentially treating prosthetic devices to reduce the risk of infection.

DIAGNOSIS

Clinically Infected Prostheses

These are relatively easily diagnosed by the presence of virulent drainage, fever, redness, and device extrusion, all of which generally occur in the perioperative period. In addition, one may see clinical infection develop any time during the life span of a prosthetic device, and this can occur in periods of 1 to 2 years after the implantation. While it is our belief that this represents activation of a subclinical infection, nonetheless, when manifested by overt clinical problems, it will have to be dealt with aggressively. The organism usually causing the infection and that will culture from the drainage is *Staphylococcus epidermidis*; seen to a lesser extent are a variety of gram-negative organisms, particularly in those individuals who were incontinent of their urine at the time of implantation. When there is drainage from the wound, culture is most useful in identifying the organisms responsible for the problem.

Subclinically Infected Prostheses

Staphylococcus epidermidis is a bacterium that infrequently associated with virulent infections; it has the ability to grow on a surface, such as silicone, enveloped in a mucous coat that is impermeable to antibiotics. As noted, this organism is responsible for most infections of prosthetic devices implanted in humans (1–8,11,18). This mucous coating, in which the microbe envelopes itself, can sustain the bacterium indefinitely, even in the face of antibiotics to which it may normally be sensitive. The cardinal feature of this subclinical infection is chronic intermittent pain; on some occasions subclinical infection progresses to an infection that is clinically quite apparent and may even lead to device extrusion.

It is also important to emphasize another point in making the diagnosis of an infected prosthesis: if the device is moving through the tissue, usually resulting in migration towards the tip of the penis, it is most likely because it is infected, not because the device is too long. This is easily recognized, since the device that is migrating frequently has significant pain associated with it. Even though the patient may have two implants, only one may be infected. Recognition of the fact that device pain and migration reflect an infectious problem is critical because this situation may be corrected. However, it may not necessarily be corrected by putting in a shorter device or exchanging a semirigid device for an inflatable one unless the infection is resolved.

THERAPY

In the event the acute infection is associated with extensive tissue involvement and fever, especially in a diabetic patient, there may be no choice but to remove the device and treat the individual with appropriate antibiotic therapy. It is not always necessary, however, to treat the acutely infected device by removing it. If there is not extensive tissue involvement, but only drainage from the prosthesis, it is possible to treat the individual with antibiotic therapy (appropriate for the organisms cultured from drainage) to convert the overtly infected prosthetic device to one that is subclinically infected. If antibiotic therapy relieves the fever, pain, and discharge, it is then possible to perform a device exchange, replacing the infected device with an uninfected one and thereby salvaging the implant.

It has been documented that one can exchange an infected device for an uninfected device (10,12). We believe that this is possible because the bacteria are on the device surface and not free in the tissue or in the tissue fluid between the device and the capsule that the body produces surrounding an implant. In theory, since this may be the case, one can remove the infected silicone prosthesis and replace it with an uninfected one. One does not have to delay the exchange. It can be done at the same surgery. We have been approximately 90% successful in this endeavor (10). It is also possible to resolve the infection with prolonged antibiotic therapy (10). It is recommended that before surgery is performed, a trial of antibiotic therapy be used, and then, if it is not successful, device exchange be attempted.

Oral Therapy

For those patients who have the diagnosis of a chronically infected prosthesis, it is worthwhile to attempt long-term drug therapy prior to performing device removal. The theory behind this is that although the organisms that are imbedded in a biofilm on the surface of the device are relatively metabolically inactive, they are not totally inactive. They will intermittently need to ingest nutrients, at which time they may also take in antibiotics. Antibiotics should be started, and if pain is suppressed by the treatment after several weeks, then therapy should be continued for at least a total of 10 to 12 weeks. If this fails to resolve the problem, surgical exchange should be considered. A major problem is difficulty in finding an oral agent that is successful at treating infection with *Staphylococcus epidermidis*.

We have found two drugs that have sometimes been successful in clearing infections. A fluoroquinolone such as ciprofloxacin has been the most successful, with perhaps 60% of the device infections being responsive to its use. We use 500 mg twice a day for 10 to 12 weeks. Cephalosporins have also been successful in our experience at controlling infection, and we have used cephalexin or cephradine 500 mg four times a day for the same period of time. However, this treatment is perhaps successful in only 25–30% of the cases. The most important sign of a successful response is reduction of pain, which takes between 1 and 3 weeks. A trial of both drugs is recommended if the first attempt is unsuccessful, since the infections are relatively indolent.

EXCHANGE PROTOCOL

Clinically Infected Prostheses

For the device that is associated with fever, erythema, and possibly drainage, it is important to treat the infection aggressively with systemic antibiotic therapy until these clinical signs resolve. Then the exchange is conducted as described below.

Subclinically Infected Prostheses

The protocol recommended is that the patient be placed on systemic antibiotic therapy for 24 to 49 hours before the device is removed. The best drug to utilize is vancomycin (250 mg IV every 12 hours) as it has excellent activity against *Staphylococcus epidermidis*. Treatment should be started on an outpatient basis prior to surgery to reduce the overall cost. The infected prosthesis should be removed and the capsule of the space in which the device was located irrigated with a combination of vancomycin and protamine (1 g vancomycin plus 50 mg protamine in 500 ml of sterile water). The cavity should be irrigated with a pediatric feeding tube and without power irrigation to prevent any damage to the capsule or extravasation of the material. It is only necessary to have a film of the solution left inside the cavity to help prevent possible recurrence of infection. We have been 90% successful at such exchanges in resolving the infection, and similar results have been suggested by others (10,12). Postoperatively the individual should be maintained on vancomycin therapy (250 to 500 mg IV every 12 hours) for approximately 1 week. This may be done on an outpatient basis.

PROPHYLAXIS

The experimental rodent model indicates the possibility of preventing device infection by using vancomycin and protamine during the surgical procedure. We now routinely irrigate the surgical site several times after the device is in place with a combination of vancomycin and protamine sulfate. We mix 1 g of vancomycin with 50 mg of protamine in 500 ml of sterile water. The device is initially soaked in the solution, and the wound is irrigated several times during the procedure and at the end of the procedure. Although very effective at preventing infection in rodents, to date we have no human data to suggest whether or not this is effective.

CONCLUSION

With the improvement of knowledge concerning infection of surgical implants by *Staphylococcus epidermidis*, new techniques have been developed to help the clinician reduce this problem. It is possible that the incidence of device infection can be reduced by irrigating the wound with a combination of vancomycin and protamine sulfate at the time of surgical implantation, as demonstrated in experimental models. If infections do develop, they may be controlled by prolonged oral (or systemic) antibiotic therapy or exchange of the implant with another, uninfected one.

REFERENCES

1. Dickinson GM, Bisno AL. Infections associated with indwelling devices. Concepts of pathogenesis: infections associated with intravascular devices. *Antimicrob Agents Chemother* 1989;33:602–607.
2. Schmitt DD, Bandyk DF, Pequet AJ, Malangoni MA, Towne JB. Mucin production by Staphylococcus epidermidis: a virulence factor promoting adherence to vascular grafts. *Arch Surg* 1986;121:89–95.
3. Slaughter L, Morris JE, Starr A. Prosthetic valvular endocarditis: a 12 year review. *Circulation* 1973;47:1319–1326.
4. Bayston R, Penny SR. Excessive production of mucoid substance in staphylococcus SIIA: a possible factor in colonization of Holter shunts. *Dev Med Child Neurol Suppl* 1972;27:25–28.
5. Bandyk DF, Berni GA, Thiele BL, Towne JB. Aortofemoral graft infection due to Staphylococcus epidermidis. *Arch Surg* 1984;119:102–108.
6. Marrie TJ, Nelligan J, Costerton JW. A scanning and transmission electron microscopic study of an infected endocardial pacemaker lead. *Circulation* 1982;66:1339–1341.
7. Franson TR, Sheth NK, Rose HD, Sohnle PG. Scanning electron microscopy of bacteria adherent to intravascular catheters. *J Clin Microbiol* 1984;20:500–505.
8. Gristina AG, Costerton JW, McGanity PLJ. Bacteria-laden biofilms: a hazard to orthopedic prostheses. *Infect Surg* 1984;3:655.
9. Kaufman JJ, Linder A, Raz S. Complications of penile prosthesis surgery for impotence. *J Urol* 1982;128:1192–1194.
10. Parsons CL, Stein PC, Dobke MK, Virden CP, Frank DH. Diagnosis and therapy of subclinically infected prostheses. *Surg Gynecol Obstet* 1993;177:504–506.
11. Nickel JC, Heaton J, Morales A, Costerton JW. Bacterial biofilm in persistent penile prosthesis-associated infection. *J Urol* 1986;135:586–588.
12. Furlow WL, Goldwasser B. Salvage of the eroded inflatable penile prosthesis: a new concept. *J Urol* 1987;138:312–314.
13. Lilly JD, Parsons CL. Bladder surface glycosaminoglycans is a human epithelial permeability barrier. *Surg Gynecol Obstet* 1990;171:493–496.
14. Parsons CL, Lilly JD, Stein PC. Epithelial dysfunction in non-bacterial cystitis (interstitial cystitis). *J Urol* 1991;145:732–735.
15. Parsons CL, Boychuk D, Jones S, Hurst R, Callahan H. Bladder surface glycosaminoglycans: an epithelial permeability barrier. *J Urol* 1990;143:139–142.
16. Teichman JMH, Stein PC, Parsons CL. Quaternary amine (protamine sulfate) is bactericidal to Staphylococcus epidermidis. *J Infect Dis* 1993;167:1500–1501.
17. Teichman JMH, Abraham VE, Stein PC, Parsons CL. Protamine sulfate and vancomycin are synergistic against Staphylococcus epidermidis prosthesis infections in vivo. *J Urol* 1994;152:213–216.
18. Christensen GD, Simpson WA, Bisno AL, Beachey EH. Adherence of slime-producing strains of Staphylococcus epidermidis to smooth surfaces. *Infect Immun* 1982;37:318–326.

Antibiotic Therapy in Urology,
edited by S. Grant Mulholland, M.D.,
Lippincott-Raven Publishers, Philadelphia © 1996.

Chapter 8

Pharmacologic Treatment of Genitourinary Fungal Infections

†Gilbert J. Wise and ‡Yefim R. Sheynkin

Division of Urology, Maimonides Medical Center, Brooklyn, New York 11219;
†SUNY Health Science Center of Brooklyn, Brooklyn, New York 11203;
‡Coney Island Hospital, Brooklyn, New York 11235

INTRODUCTION

Fungal infection in the urologic patient is uncommon in clinical practice. Nevertheless, the occurrence of genitourinary fungal infection or systemic infection involving the urologic patient has become more prevalent (1). The reasons for this are multiple. There is a rapidly expanding pool of immunocompromised patients who are at risk for such infections.

Certain fungi, notably *Candida*, *Aspergillus*, and *Cryptococcus*, are opportunistic—that is, they have an increased predilection for the critically ill or immunocompromised patient (2). Broad-spectrum antibiotics and indwelling urinary catheters increase the patient's vulnerability to candiduria (3). An increased incidence of candidal infection has been noted in patients with leukemia, lymphoma, and solid tumors (4). Other contributing factors for opportunistic fungal infection include diabetes mellitus, steroids or immunosuppressive therapy, and acquired immune suppressive disease. Patients receiving peritoneal dialysis may develop candidal peritonitis (5). Transplant patients are another group who have an increased vulnerability to secondary fungal infection (6). *Blastomyces*, *Coccidioides*, and *Histoplasma* are indigenous to the environment and may cause infection that affects the genitourinary system. *Mucor*, *Penicillium*, *Geotrichum*, and *Paecilomyces* have until recent years been unusual causes of clinical infection, but in the era of the immunocompromised patient these fungi can cause systemic and genitourinary disease (1).

Fungi are a distinctive group of microorganisms that differ from bacteria in morphology, cell function, and biochemistry (7,8). For these rea-

TABLE 1. *Pharmacotherapy of genitourinary fungal infection in immunocompetent adults*[a]

Disease	Site	Drug	Dose	Duration
Aspergillosis	Kidney	Amphotericin B	1.5 mg/kg/d IV ± 50 μg/ml >40 ml/h irrigation	6–18 wk
		Itraconazole	200 mg PO bid	1 y
Blastomycosis	Prostate	Ketoconazole	400 mg PO daily	>1 mo
		Amphotericin B	1–2.3 g total dose IV	3 mo
	Epididymis	Ketoconazole	400 mg PO daily	1 y
Candidiasis	Glans penis (balanitis)	Nystatin, clotrimazole	Topical cream or ointment	Not specified
		Ketoconazole	PO	Not specified
	Vagina	Nystatin	100,000 units intravaginally	14 d
		Miconazole	100 mg intravaginally	7 d
		Clotrimazole	100 mg intravaginally	7 d
		Ketoconazole	400 mg/d × 14 d, then 100 mg/d	6 mo
	Bladder	Amphotericin B	50 μg/ml >50 ml/h irrigation	4–14 d
		Miconazole	50 μg/ml >40 ml/h irrigation	5 d
		Fluconazole	400 mg loading, then 200 mg/d PO	14 d
	Kidney	Amphotericin B	1 g total dose IV ± 50 μg/ml < 40 ml/h irrigation	Not specified
Coccidioidomycosis	Kidney	Amphotericin B ± flucytosine	IV ± PO	Not specified
	Prostate	Amphotericin B	2.5 g total dose IV	4 mo
	Bladder	Amphotericin B + ketoconazole	2 g total dose IV + 200 mg PO daily	1 y
Cryptococcosis	Prostate	Amphotericin B	1–3.4 g total IV dose	Not specified
		Flucytosine	100–150 mg/d/kg body weight (normal renal function)	4–6 wk
		Fluconazole	200 mg/d	2–6 mo
Geotrichosis	Vagina	Nystatin	100,000 units intravaginally	14 d
Histoplasmosis		Amphotericin B	IV	Not specified
		Itraconazoale	PO	Not specified
		Ketoconazole	PO	Not specified
Phycomycosis		Amphotericin B	1 g total dose IV	1 mo
Sporotrichosis		Amphotericin B + flucytosine	IV + PO	Not specified
		Itraconazole	PO	Not specified
Torulopsis	Kidney	Ketoconazole	800 mg/d PO	7 mo
		Amphotericin B	700 mg total dose IV	Not specified
		Flucytosine	500 mg QID PO	8 wk
	Bladder	Amphotericin B + flucytosine	15–30 mg/d irrigation + 20–100 mg/d PO	30 d + 6–8 wk

[a]Entries represent known dosage and guidelines only. Specific therapy must be tailored to each patient, with drug selection, dose, and duration of treatment determined by sensitivity testing, metabolic considerations, and clinical and laboratory evidence of improvement.

sons, they do not respond to the antibiotics that are effective against bacteria but require a special group of antimicrobial agents (9).

This chapter reviews the pharmacologic agents necessary in the management of genitourinary fungal infections. Guidelines for the pharmacotherapy of genitourinary fungal infections have been outlined and depicted in Table 1. A concise overview of indications for treatment is presented.

INDICATIONS FOR PHARMACOLOGIC TREATMENT

Indications for pharmacologic intervention include persistent funguria and/or positive culture sites, i.e., wound, gastrointestinal tract, or blood. Antifungal therapy should be considered in the critically ill patient with fever in whom a putative cause cannot be clearly defined. The diagnosis of invasive fungal infections is often difficult to establish. Blood cultures are often negative, and the fungus may be difficult to identify from the infected site. Serologic tests have been utilized to diagnosis systemic infection caused by *Candida*. Laboratory studies have included precipitin, enzyme immunoassay, and radio immunoassay of antibody formation to fungal antigen (10,11). In the critically ill patient, immune response may be muted, so antibody titers may not be detected. Recent studies suggest that the presence of candidal antigenemia may provide a new diagnostic tool for candidal infection (12,13). However, none of these methods has gained wide clinical use. Polymerase chain reaction (PCR) has been utilized for the detection of *C. albicans* DNA. This very sensitive method can circumvent the problems of slow-growing fungal cultures and delay in diagnosis and treatment (14). These diagnostic tools are still experimental, so the clinician must continue to utilize the classic methods of diagnosis of infection: clinical awareness, standard laboratory procedures, and radiographic and endoscopic modalities.

PHARMACOLOGIC THERAPY

Amphotericin B

The actinomycete *Streptomyces nodosus* was found to have fungicidal properties; these observations led to the development of antifungal agents known as the polyene antibiotics that bind to the sterol cell membranes and disrupt the integrity of the cellular components (15). The polyene consist of variety of agents whose common chemical structure is characterized by macrolide rings formed by internal esters or lactones and bearing several hydroxyl groups. The polyene rings vary from 26 to 28 carbon atoms, with biologic activity dependent on the conjugated double bonds and molecular size (Fig. 1). The polyene antibiotics can be either fungicidal or fungistatic depending on the concentration, molecular structure, and ability to bind to fungal cell wall membranes.

Most significantly, the polyene antibiotics pose problems with solubility, stabilization, absorption, and toxicity. For these reasons, only amphotericin B (amp B) has proved to be suitable for systemic use.

Nystatin is chemically similar to the amphotericin B; because of poor solubility it is used primarily as a topical antifungal agent. It has had limited use as a genitourinary irrigant. Amphotericin B, in addition to its an-

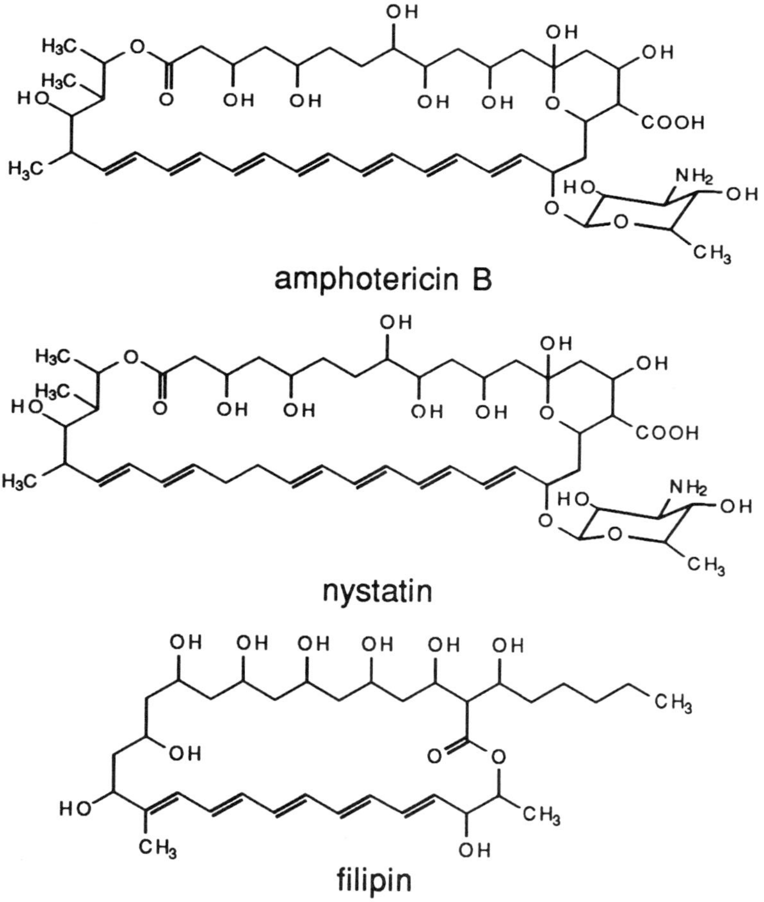

FIG. 1. Chemical structure of the polyene antibiotics. (From Medoff and Kobayashi, ref. 9, with permission.)

tifungal effects, has immunopotentiation properties that enhance the number of antibody-producing cells in the spleen and lymph nodes of experimental animals (9).

Amphotericin B is still considered the gold standard of treatment of invasive or systemic fungal infection. For this reason, the knowledge of its use is important in the management of serious genitourinary fungal infections. Because of the difficulties encountered in preparation and use, there may be a tendency on the part of many physicians not to use amp B; however, delay in its use may adversely affect the patient's outcome. Amp B is a bile salt complex that forms a colloidal suspension when hydrated. It is used as an intravenous agent suspended in dextrose and water and as a genitourinary irrigant when suspended in water. The mixture of amp B and saline or other electrolyte-containing material results in a cloudy suspension wherein the colloid aggregates (16).

Amp B is not readily absorbed from the gastrointestinal tract; it must be given by the intravenous route for a systemic effect. Amp B has been given orally to decrease fungal colonization in the gastrointestinal tract. The effectiveness of amp B in association with broad-spectrum antibiotics to reduce gastrointestinal colonization has not been clearly documented (15). Following intravenous administration, amp B is distributed in the liver, spleen, kidney, muscle, and skin; distribution is poor in the cerebrospinal and peritoneal fluid (15,17). Approximately 10% of administered amp B is retained in the plasma, with 90% bound to lipoprotein. The drug is excreted in the urine slowly; hemodialysis does not affect plasma drug levels. It is estimated that the initial half-life of amp B is 24 hours, and the drug can last as long as 15 days following single dose. Although renal function accounts for small proportion of amp B clearance, the kidneys can be vulnerable to amp B toxicity; hence, drug dosage should be modified in the patients with underlying renal disease. Blood urea nitrogen, creatinine, and serum electrolytes, including potassium and magnesium, should be monitored closely during systemic therapy.

Systemic Administration of Amphotericin B

Prior to use, amp B should be given as a test dose of 1 ml dissolved in 50 to 100 ml of 5% dextrose and water and administered intravenously over 20 to 30 minutes. If there is no adverse reaction, then treatment can be started at 0.25 mg/kg body weight in 500 ml of 5% dextrose and administered over 2 to 6 hours. Subsequently, increments yielding 0.3 mg/kg, 0.35 mg/kg, and 0.4 mg/kg should be given until the final dose of 0.5 mg/kg is achieved (18). The maximum dose of 0.5 mg/kg (35 mg/day for a 70-kg man) can be attained within 5 to 7 days provided the patient has no adverse reaction to the drug administration. In cases of severe infection, higher doses of 1 mg/kg body weight may be necessary. Simultaneous administration of corticosteroid may be utilized to minimize the "anaphylactic" reaction often associated with the intravenous administration of amp B.

Controlled studies that document the effectiveness of amphotericin B in the treatment of fungal infection of the genitourinary system have not been reported. Based on its use in systemic fungal infections, amp B has become the drug of choice for the treatment of invasive genitourinary fungal infections.

Amphotericin B as a Genitourinary Irrigant

In 1960, amphotericin B suspension was documented as an effective antifungal genitourinary irrigant in the management of localized fungal candidal infection of the bladder (19). Although the drug insert does not describe its use as a genitourinary irrigant, it has become common practice to use this agent, which has demonstrated better than 90% effectiveness in the treatment of localized bladder infection (20). For use as a genitourinary irrigant, amp B is suspended in 1 ml sterile water, which provides a concentration of 50 μg/ml. This exceeds the minimal inhibitory concentration (MIC) for most known fungal species that affect the genitourinary tract. The irrigant is then administered to the bladder via three-way catheter or via urethral catheter and suprapubic tube over 24 hours for 5 to 7 days. A repeated course may be necessary. Another method utilizes amphotericin B suspension of 10 μg/ml instilled into the bladder for 60 to 90 minutes (21). Amp B has been used as a genitourinary irrigant via nephrostomy tube in the management of upper tract and candidal infection. In many cases, amp B has been used in conjunction with surgical removal of fungal material from collecting system (22). Amp B suspension has been useful in neonates who develop the fungal infection with obstruction to the upper tract. In these cases, the dosage has been modified from 10 μg/kg/hour to 2 μg/kg/hour (23). Amp B doses as high as 100 μg/ml have also been utilized in neonates without ill effect (24). As amp B has been known to lose 26% activity within 3 days when exposed to room temperature and light, daily preparation of this agent and covering the suspension bottle and irrigant tubing with aluminum foil to minimize light and heat exposure are advised. Amp B suspension can be stored in the refrigerator for 1 week without adverse impact (25). Amp B genitourinary irrigations have not resulted in systemic absorption of the drug; no adverse effect has been noted from the use of Amp B as a genitourinary irrigant (20).

Amp B in the Treatment of Fungal Peritonitis

Fungal peritonitis may occur in patients who have a ruptured abdominal viscus or require peritoneal dialysis, or after exploratory laparotomy (26,27). Treatment of fungal peritonitis includes surgical drainage and systemic treatment with amp B and flucytosine. Peritoneal lavage with amp B has been utilized. Initially, a test dose of 10 mg of amp B suspended in 5% dextrose and water with 25 mg of hydrocortisone is inserted into the peritoneal cavity for 30 minutes. If there is no adverse reaction, then the patient receives subsequent dosages of 25 mg amp B at 48-hour intervals. Serum levels of amp B range from 15–30% of ascitic fluid levels (28). Fungal peritonitis is serious, and hence aggressive systemic therapy as well as intraperitoneal irrigations with amp B are advocated. In patients on peritoneal dialysis, the intraperitoneal catheter may have to be removed to resolve the intraperitoneal fungal infection.

Indications for Systemic Use of Amphotericin B

The urologist may rarely use systemic amp B. Chronic funguria from candidal species in the upper tracts or the bladder may be resolved by appropriate drainage and the use of antifungal genitourinary irrigants (2). When the fungal infection becomes invasive and/or disseminated, then systematic amp B is indicated. Genitourinary aspergillosis, cryptococcosis, coccidioidomycosis, histoplasmosis, blastomycosis, and other noncandidal fungal infections require 4 to 16 weeks of therapy with a minimum total dosage of 1,000 mg amp B. In genitourinary candidal infections, modified doses of amp B of 400 mg given over 2 to 3 weeks may be sufficient (21).

Liposomal Amphotericin B

Administration of amphotericin B is not without adverse effect, notably renal toxicity and electrolyte imbalance. Newer pharmacologic techniques offer the prospect of delivering the drug to the infected tissue without the potential for serious adverse effect. Investigational studies indicate that liposomal amphotericin B fulfills two criteria, namely, high tissue levels and lessened toxicity. Liposomes are microscopic "fat bubbles" that contain bilayered phospholipid membranes. Encapsulation of drugs within the liposomes has provided a new modality with which to deliver drug to specific areas, such as the reticuloendothelial system, spleen, lung, lymph nodes, and bone marrow. Liposomal amphotericin B is much less toxic than other forms of amphotericin B, particularly in regard to renal damage.

Clinical studies to date are limited but indicate that liposomal amp B preparation is efficacious in the treatment of systemic fungal infections (29). One study reported on 126 patients with 137 episodes of fungal infections treated at 43 investigational centers. Fungi were eradicated in 65% of evaluated cases (30). Liposomal amp B has been used with success in the treatment of four patients with urinary tract infection caused by *Candida albicans*. Urine became negative within 4 days of treatment (31). Liposomal amp B may provide another modality with which to treat urinary fungal infections.

Amphotericin B Lipid Complex

Another amphotericin B agent utilizes a lipid complex composed of phospholipid dimyrisoyl phosphatidylcholine. This complex (ABLC) achieves good tissue concentration without adverse effect of amphotericin B. To date there are no clinical studies that document its use in genitourinary infections (29).

Therapy of Genitourinary Fungal Infections with 5-Fluorocytosine (Flucytosine)

5-Fluorocytosine (flucytosine, 5-FC) (Ancobon; Roche) was synthesized in 1957 (32). Developed as a potential antitumor agent (it is an analog of 5-fluorouracil), it proved ineffective in the treatment of tumors in animal models; serendipity indicated that the drug is inhibitory to fungal growth. 5-Fluorocytosine is converted to 5-fluorouracil (5-FU) by cytosine deaminase, which is present in some fungal species but is absent or present in low concentrations in mammalian cells (9). 5-FU is then converted to 5-fluorodoxyuridine monophosphate, which adversely affects fungal protein and DNA synthesis (9) (Fig. 2). Fungal resistance to 5-FC has been attributed to either lack of cytosine deaminase or uridine monophosphate pyrophosphorylase, which control the metabolism of 5-FU. Flucytosine is fluorinated pyrimidine. Its molecular weight is 129.1 and it is readily absorbed by the gastrointestinal tract and widely distributed in a volume approximating the total body water (15,33).

There is little binding to plasma proteins, and the drug is primarily excreted by glomerular filtration. Serum half-life ranges from 3 to 5 hours, and there is good penetration into the cerebrospinal fluid and other body fluids. Serum concentrations may reach as high as 70 to 80 μg/ml within 1 to 2 hours after a dose of 37.5 mg/kg. This far exceeds the MIC of 5-FC-sensitive fungi. The drug is excreted unchanged by filtration and may reach urine levels of 200 to 500 μg/ml. As the primary method of excretion is renal, the dosage must be modified in the presence of

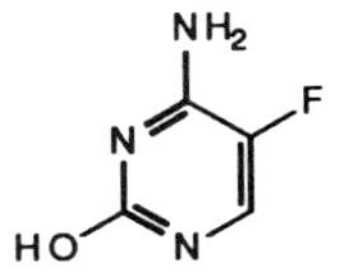

FIG. 2. Chemical structure of flucytosine. (From Medoff and Kobayashi, ref. 9, with permission.)

renal disease. When first introduced, 5-FC was administered in doses of 50 mg/kg. Presently, a dose of 100 to 150 mg/kg is advised (34,35). Flucytosine can be given every 6 hours; however, in the presence of renal insufficiency, dosage should be modified in proportion to degree of renal compromise. With creatinine clearance of 25 to 40 ml/min, the drug would be given every 12 hours, whereas with a creatinine clearance of 12.5 to 25 ml/min the interval would be increased to 24 hours; if creatinine clearance is less than 12.5 ml, one dose should be given followed by assessment of serum levels of 5-FC. Flucytosine can be cleared by dialysis, so renal failure should not preclude its use when the drug is clinically indicated (9).

Whenever possible, treatment should be monitored by assessment of serum levels of 5-FC correlated with in vitro evaluation of MIC and minimal fungicidal concentration (MFC). A serum level at four times the in vitro MICs has been utilized to monitor the treatment in patients with genitourinary candidiasis (35).

Flucytosine induces both inhibitory and fungicidal effects primarily on candidal species, including *C. glabrata* (also known as *Torulopsis glabrata*), and *Cryptococcus* (2). Success has been noted in occasional cases of *Aspergillus* infection. No documented effect has been noted in other fungal infections of the genitourinary system, such as blastomycosis, histoplasmosis, and coccidioidomycosis.

Adverse Effects of Flucytosine

Flucytosine's adverse effects may include nausea, vomiting, diarrhea, and enterocolitis. Abnormalities in liver function have been noted in 5% of patients (15). Bone marrow depression may occur with the development of anemia, leukopenia, and thrombocytopenia. These toxic manifestations resolve with stoppage of drug, although one case of aplastic anemia has been associated with 5-FC (36). The drug is contraindicated in pregnancy, although it has been given to a pregnant woman during the second trimester without adverse effect in the fetus (37). In some series, successful management of urinary candidal infection has been reported to vary from 50–90% (34,35,38).

Primary resistance to drug may occur in 10% of cases infected with *C. albicans* but may be as high as 30% with other candidal species. Secondary resistance was noted to occur in 6.2% of patients within 7 to 10 days of treatment.

Indications for Use

Flucytosine can be utilized as an alternate treatment in patients with persistent candiduria that does not resolve with other modalities, i.e., fluconazole (to be discussed) or amphotericin B irrigations.

Flucytosine can be used in those patients who have not only persistent candiduria but also evidence of fungal infection at other sites, such as oropharynx and/or wound. When used alone, 5-FC should be given in doses of 150 mg/kg provided there is a normal renal function. For example, in 70-kg patient, the dose would be 70 × 150 or 10.5 g/day. Insofar as flucytosine is available in 250- or 500-ml capsules, the 70-kg adult would be given 10.5 g divided by 0.5 or 21 capsules per day in divided doses: 6 capsules after breakfast, 5 capsules after lunch and dinner, and 5 capsules at bedtime. If the patient develops nausea, then the dosage may be modified accordingly, or a smaller number of capsules given at more frequent intervals.

With elderly or dysphagic patients, the capsule may be opened and medication placed in food or given via tube feedings. Flucytosine can be given to pediatric patients; for children who weigh less than 50 kg, a daily dosage schedule of 4,500 mg/m^2 body surface is advocated (39,40).

Cryptococcal infection can affect the prostate and kidney (2). Flucytosine may be useful in those patients with cryptococcal genitourinary disease.

Combination Therapy

The utilization of systemic amphotericin B in combination with 5-FC has been advocated in the treatment of severe cryptococcal infections, particularly cryptococcal meningitis (9). Amphotericin B in lower and less toxic dosages is believed to affect the fungal cell membrane, thereby facilitating the entrance of 5-FC into intracellular sites. However, there have been no documented studies on the effect of combined amphotericin B and flucytosine in the treatment of invasive genitourinary fungal infections.

Flucytosine has not been advocated as readily as primary treatment in recent years for a variety reasons: (a) the emergence of resistance strains;

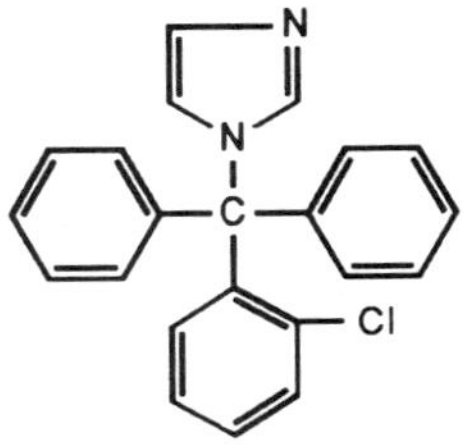

clotrimazole

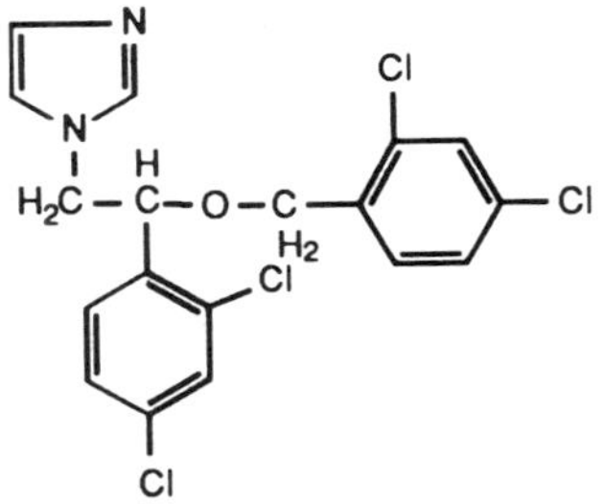

miconazole

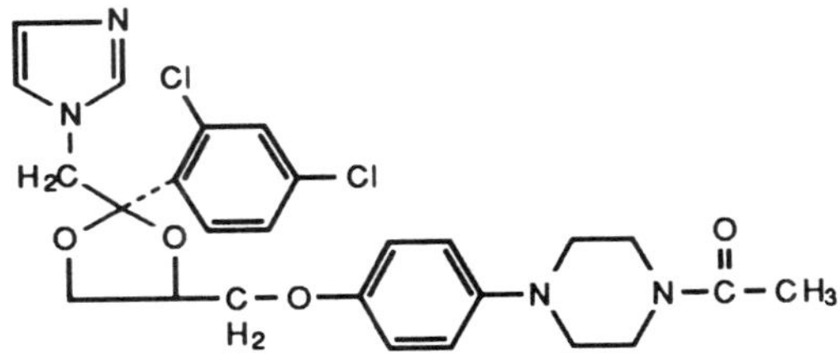

ketoconazole

FIG. 3. Chemical structure of imidazoles. (From Medoff and Kobayashi, ref. 9, with permission.)

(b) the introduction of a newer class of antifungal agents, the triazoles, which include fluconazole; (c) the availability of antifungal genitourinary irrigants in the hospital setting; and (d) 5-FC's adverse effects on the hematopoietic system and liver.

Imidazoles

The imidazoles include clotrimazole, a topical agent; miconazole, which has been used both intravenously and as a genitourinary irrigant; and ketoconazole, which can be administered by mouth for systemic infection (9)

(Fig. 3). Another imidazole, econazole, is available in the United States as a topical antifungal agent (41).

The primary mechanism of action of the imidazoles is interference with fungal ergosterol metabolism, which alters cell membrane integrity and thus disrupts cellular metabolism (42). Cytochrome P-450 of yeast is also affected by miconazole and ketoconazole (9,15).

Miconazole

Miconazole (Monistat; Janssen Laboratories) is available in 20-ml ampules at a drug concentration of 10 mg/ml (200 mg/ampule). This drug can be used intravenously by dissolving in 200 ml of either normal saline or 5% dextrose and water. For therapeutic effect, dosage may vary from 200 to 1,200 mg given every 8 hours (42). The drug has been reported effective in a variety of fungi that can infect the genitourinary system, such as *Candida*, *Aspergillus*, and *Histoplasma*. Toxic reactions have been noted and may include anaphylaxis, cardiac arrhythmias, fever, chills, nausea, anemia, and liver abnormalities. For these reasons, an initial test dose of 200 mg should be given prior to starting the patient on therapy (18). Intravenous administration can yield serum levels of 6 μg/ml; the short serum half-life causes concentrations to drop rapidly to 0.1 to 0.6 μg/ml, so administration every 8 hours is advised. Ninety percent of the drug is bound to serum albumin. The drug is primarily metabolized by the liver, and there is minimal renal excretion. As miconazole is poorly excreted into the urine, it has a limited role (when given intravenously) in the management of primary urinary fungal infections (42). In view of its toxicity, its ineffectiveness against urinary infection, and the availability of new drugs, miconazole has no role as a systemically administered agent in the treatment of invasive fungal infection. Miconazole should be utilized only as a genitourinary antifungal irrigant for the treatment of localized infection.

Utilization of miconazole as a genitourinary irrigant has proved successful in patients with candidal colonization or noninvasive infection (43). Miconazole has been effective in a small series of patients with persistent candiduria. Dosage has been 50 mg or 100 mg diluted in a liter of sterile water and given over 24 hours for 5 to 7 days. The irrigating solution is prepared by dissolving a 200-mg ampule of miconazole in 4 l of sterile water, which then can be stored at room temperature. Unlike amp B, miconazole is stable at ambient temperature. The cost of miconazole treatment is 25% that of amphotericin B when used as a genitourinary irrigant.

For stability, miconazole suspension must be prepared in rigid nonpolyvinyl plastic containers.

Ketoconazole

Ketoconazole is readily absorbed into circulation from the gastrointestinal tract, and thus it can be administered orally. However, absorption is limited if the patient has achlorhydria or uses antacids, cimetidine, or ranitidine (42). The drug is available in either 200- or 400-mg tablets (15). A 400-mg dose can achieve serum levels of 1.8 to 7.8 μg/ml, which exceeds the in vitro MIC of many candidal species (including *Torulopsis*), *Coccidioides*, *Cryptococcus*, *Aspergillus*, *Histoplasma*, and *Blastomyces* (44). Because of its poor renal excretion, ketoconazole does not reach adequate urinary drug levels sufficient to inhibit many fungal species.

Ketoconazole's adverse effects include headaches and skin rashes, but its most significant impact is on liver metabolism, with elevation of serum triglycerides and potential liver toxicity. Ketoconazole affects mammalian steroid metabolism, with impairment of androgen synthesis. For this reason it has been utilized in the management of prostatic carcinoma (45). An initial dose of 400 mg/day with gradual increase to 800 mg/day in divided doses is recommended. Therapy may be required for many months, in disseminated coccidioidomycosis for 12 months or longer (18). In pediatric cases with systemic fungal disease, ketoconazole in daily divided doses of 7 to 10 mg/kg has been utilized with good results (46). Hepatotoxicity appears to be more prevalent in younger children (47). Transplant patients are prone to secondary fungal infection. Imidazoles should be given cautiously in those patients requiring cyclosporin, as there is a drug interaction between cyclosporin and the imidazoles in which ketoconazole increases serum cyclosporin levels (48).

Triazoles

In recent years two new antifungal agents, the triazoles, have been developed. The major structural difference is three nitrogen atoms in the azole ring, compared with two in the imidazoles (Fig. 4).

Fluconazole

Fluconazole's mode of action is similar to that of ketoconazole, inhibition of synthesis of ergosterol, which is a component of the fungal cell membrane. The step required to convert 14-αmethylsterol to ergosterol depends on cytochrome P-450 activation, which is inhibited by the imidazole moiety (49). Fluconazole has good water solubility, which results in high levels of urinary excretion.

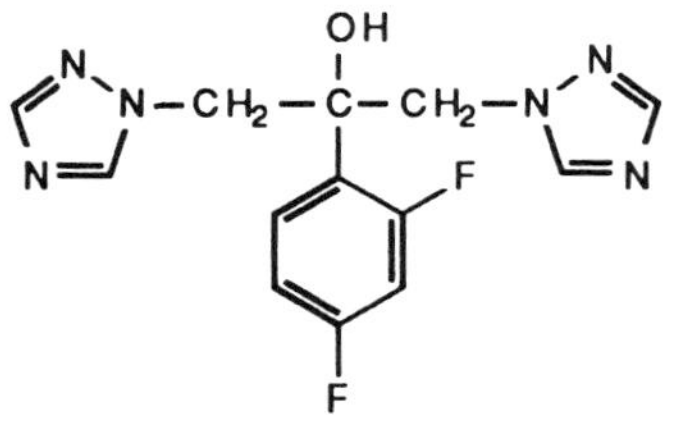

FIG. 4. Chemical structure of fluconazole.

In animal model experiments, fluconazole has been efficacious in the treatment of aspergillosis, blastomycosis, candidiasis, coccidioidomycosis, and histoplasmosis. The drug has excellent absorption from the gastrointestinal tract—better than 90%. Unlike ketoconazole, fluconazole is not dependent on gastric acidity. Peak serum concentrations are reached in 2 hours. There is minimal protein binding (12%), and the drug is metabolically stable, with renal excretion accounting for 80% of elimination. Plasma half-life is approximately 30 hours (50,51). Rifampin decreases the half-life of fluconazole, but to a lesser degree than it does with ketoconazole. There is minimal interaction with warfarin, phenytoin, and cyclosporin (50). Fluconazole does not inhibit steroidogenesis to the same degree as ketoconazole. The dosage of fluconazole should be modified in the presence of renal failure. The drug can be administered in patients undergoing hemodialysis.

Fluconazole should be administered as a loading dose of 400 mg the first day and 200 mg for an additional 13 days. In patients with renal insufficiency (serum creatinine :3.0 mg), fluconazole dosage should be reduced accordingly, to a loading dose of 100 mg and a daily dose of 50 mg. Fluconazole may be given by intravenously at 200 mg/day in the critically ill or postsurgical patient who cannot take the drug orally.

In two studies involving 22 patients with leukemia with chronic disseminated candidiasis documented by culture and/or liver biopsy, 11 patients (50%) had putative renal involvement as indicated by CT (50,52). Prior treatment with amphotericin B with or without flucytosine was unsuccessful in eradicating candidiasis in 17 (77%) patients, whereas fluconazole was successful. Two (9%) patients with candidiasis involving the kidney died.

Fluconazole was also evaluated in 24 children who had 34 episodes of candidiasis. All the patients had underlying predisposing factors, such as human immunodeficiency virus infection (8 patients), organ or bone marrow transplant (7 patients), neoplasia (5 patients), obstructive uropathy (3 patients), or neonatal age and malnutrition (1 patient) (53). Five patients had urinary infections caused by candidal species. Four

(80%) of the five urinary tract infections responded to fluconazole (6mg/kg/day; median, 12 days).

Itraconazole

Itraconazole binds to fungal cytochrome P-450, thereby inhibiting fungal capsule ergosterol biosynthesis and interfering with the 14-αdimethylation of lanosterol. Following oral administration, itraconazole achieves peak plasma levels within 1.5 to 4 hours (49). Absorption is enhanced by the presence of food in the stomach, which produces increased gastric acidity; its absorption is reduced by antacids but not H_2 blockers (54). Itraconazole is lipophilic: tissue concentrations are 2 to 3 times higher than in plasma, whereas adipose tissue concentrations are 20 times higher. The drug is metabolized in the liver and excreted primarily via the biliary system. Like the other azole compounds, itraconazole has the potential for liver toxicity. Nausea, vomiting, hypokalemia, and abnormal liver enzymes have occurred in 5–10% of patients taking 400 mg/day (55). Higher doses (600 mg/day) have been reported to cause hypotension, hypokalemia, and adrenal insufficiency.

Drugs that affect hepatic drug-metabolizing enzymes increase the metabolism of itraconazole. These include isoniazid, rifampin, phenobarbital, carbamazepine, and dilantin (56). Itraconazole may potentiate the effect and toxicity of phenytoin, cyclosporin, oral hypoglycemic drugs, warfarin, digoxin, and certain antihistamines (terfenadine and astemizole). Didanosine utilized in the treatment of patients with AIDS can interfere with the gastrointestinal absorption of itraconazole (57). Because of low urinary levels, itraconazole has limited use in the treatment of funguria. However, its ability to reach good tissue levels may make it suitable for parenchymal infection caused by a number of fungal species, such as *Candida* (including *Torulopsis*), *Cryptococcus*, *Aspergillus*, *Blastomyces*, *Coccidioides*, and *Histoplasma*.

European studies have reported on the use of itraconazole in more than 100 patients with deep fungal infections (58). Evaluation was possible in 34 patients with aspergillosis, 22 with cryptococcosis, and 1 with sporotrichosis. Predisposing factors included organ (heart) transplant, lymphoma, and AIDS. Thirty-one of 34 patients with aspergillosis had a cure or improvement with itraconazole. Twenty of 22 patients with cryptococcosis had cure or improvement with itraconazole.

None of the patients had documented genitourinary involvement. An isolated episode of hypokalemia was the only adverse effect noted. The drug appears to be well tolerated for long-term maintenance therapy.

To date there are limited clinical data on the use of itraconazole in the treatment of genitourinary fungal infections.

UNCOMMON OR EXPERIMENTAL TREATMENT MODALITIES

Alkalinization of Urine

The ideal pH for growth of *Candida* ranges from 5.1 to 6.4, which parallels that of urine pH. Alkalinization of the urine has been cited as a method of resolving candiduria. These observations appear to be anecdotal, insofar as there have been no clinical studies that have documented these findings in recent literature.

Transfer Factor

Transfer factor derived from lymphocyte lysate has been helpful in the treatment of generalized coccidioidomycosis, histoplasmosis, and chronic mucocutaneous candidiasis (59). The authors had several patients with both systemic and severe urinary candidiasis who have been helped with transfer factor. This agent is available only from research and/or blood bank laboratories.

Miscellaneous Antifungal Agents

Allylamine derivatives of naftifine have demonstrated in vitro and in vivo antifungal activity. Their mechanism of action involves fungal inhibition of ergosterol biosynthesis. These drugs are still in experimental study (60).

Oral nifuratel (a nitrofuran) had been reported effective in a small group of patients with candidal urinary tract infection; however, this agent has never gained widespread clinical use (61). Another agent, Mepartricin, a semisynthetic haptene, was reported successful in 10 of 11 immunocompromised patients with systemic candidal infection (62). Its use in genitourinary fungal infections has not been reported.

TOPICAL TREATMENT OF GENITAL FUNGAL INFECTION

A variety of topically effective drugs are available for the treatment of superficial candidal infection. Nystatin (Mycostatin) has been the standard topical agent. In recent years, clotrimazole or miconazole have become available in creams and vaginal inserts. Boric acid powder (placed in gelatin capsules) has been very effective in the control of vaginal infections (63). Nystatin and miconazole have been used intravaginally during pregnancy (64).

PREVENTION

Awareness of the contributory factors to genitourinary fungal infection may help in the prevention of these opportunistic infections. As indicated previously, the removal of indwelling catheters and intravenous lines and the avoidance, if possible, of multiple broad-spectrum antibiotics are advised. The use of antifungal medication has been advocated to decrease fungal colonization of the gastrointestinal tract in the hope that this would prevent dissemination to other organs. The oral administration of nystatin, amphotericin B, and ketoconazole has been utilized as antifungal prophylaxis in the treatment of bone marrow transplant patients (65).

Oral candidal infection (thrush) has been prevented in patients with AIDS or AIDS-related complex by the use of oral fluconazole (66). However, there have been no documented studies that cite the use of oral antifungal agents to prevent secondary genitourinary infections.

COST FACTOR

Table 2 lists the costs for antifungal therapy with various agents. These costs may vary in different locations (67). The choice of drug should be

TABLE 2. *Cost comparison of antifungal agents*

Drug	Unit cost ($)	Daily dose[a]	Cost per day ($)
Flucytosine capsules			
Ancobon 250 mg	1.01	50–150 mg/kg[b]	14.14–
Ancobon 500 mg (Roche)	1.93	(3.5–10.5 mg)	42.42
Amphotericin B 50 mg/vial			
Fungizone (Squibb)	37.06	Usually 0.5 mg/kg[b]	37.06
Amphotericin B (Lyphomed)	38.49	(50 mg or less)	38.49
Ketoconazole 200-mg tablet			
Nizoral 200 mg (Janssen)	2.32	200–400 mg	2.32– 4.64
Miconazole 200 mg/amp			
Monistat 200 mg/amp (Janssen)	38.47	IV: 3–9 amps (600 mg–1.8 g)	115.41– 346.23
Fluconazole			
Diflucan 100 mg PO	6.88	200 mg	13.76
Diflucan 200 mg IV (Roerig)	81.25	200 mg	81.25
Itraconazole			
Sporanox 100 mg PO (Janssen)	4.92	100 mg PO	4.92

[a]The duration of the therapy for fungal infection depends on the causative agents. Therapy may be as short as 1 week or may continue for a period of weeks to months. The following are only general approximations: flucytosine, weeks to months; amphotericin B, weeks to months; ketoconazole, 1 to 4 weeks, 6 to 12 months; miconazole, 1 to 20 weeks; fluconazole, weeks to months; itraconazole, weeks to months.

[b]Daily dose calculated for 70 kg.

based on clinical, not economic, factors. The cost factors are presented to emphasize the significant economic as well as medical impact made by fungal infections.

REFERENCES

1. Wise GJ, Silver DA. Fungal infections of genitourinary system. *J Urol* 1993;149:1377–1388.
2. Wise GJ. Fungi in the genitourinary system. *AUA Update Series* 1984;23:3–8.
3. Hamory BH, Wenzel RP. Hospital associated candiduria: predisposing factors and review of the literature. *J Urol* 1978;120:444–448.
4. Horn R, Wong B, Kiehn TE. Fungemia in a cancer hospital: changing frequency, earlier onset and results of therapy. *Rev Infect Dis* 1985;7:646–655.
5. Struijk DG, Krediet RT, Boeschoten EW, et al. Antifungal treatment of Candida peritonitis in continuous ambulatory peritoneal dialysis patients. *Am J Kidney Dis* 1987;9:66–70.
6. Gallis HA, Berman RA, Cate TR, Hamilton JD, Gunnells JC, Stickel DL. Fungal infection following renal transplantation. *Arch Intern Med* 1975;135:1163.
7. Rippon JW. Characteristics of fungi. In: xxxx, eds. *Medical mycology, the pathogenic fungi and pathogenic actinomycetes.* 3rd ed. Philadelphia: WB Saunders;1988:121–153.
8. Whittaker RH. New concepts of kingdoms of organisms. *Science* 1969;163:150–160.
9. Medoff G, Kobayashi GS. Strategies in the treatment of systemic fungal infections. *N Engl J Med* 1980;302:145–155.
10. Kozinn PJ, Taschdjian CL, Goldberg PK, et al. Advances in the diagnosis of renal candidiasis. *J Urol* 1978;119:184–187.
11. deRepentigny L, Reiss E. Current trends in immunodiagnosis of candidiasis and aspergillosis. *Rev Infect Dis* 1984;6:301–312.
12. Suits T, Walters B, Wise GJ. Candidal antigenemia: a prognostic determinant in candidal urinary tract infection. *J Urol* 1989;141:1381–1384.
13. Walsh TJ, Hathorn JW, Sobel JD, Merz WG, Sanchez V, Maret SM, Buckley HR, Pfaller MA, Schaufele R, Sliva C. Detection of circulating Candida enolase by immunoassay in patients with cancer and invasive candidiasis. *New Engl J Med* 1991;324:1026–1031.
14. Buchman TG, Rossier M, Merz WG, Garache P. Detection of surgical pathogens by in vitro DNA amplification. Part I. Rapid identification of Candida albicans by in vitro amplification of fungus-specific gene. *Surgery* 1990;108:338–347.
15. Sande MA, Mandell GL. Antimicrobial agents: antifungal and antiviral agents. In: Gilman AG, ed. *The pharmacological basis of therapeutics.* 7th ed. New York: MacMillan Publishers; 1985:1219.
16. Bennett J. Chemotherapy of systemic mycoses. *N Engl J Med* 1974;290:30–32.
17. Craven PG, Ludden TM, Drutz DJ, et al. Excretion pathways of amphotericin B. *J Infect Dis* 1979;140:329–340.
18. Drugs for treatment of systemic fungal infection. *Med Lett Drugs Ther* 1986;28:41.
19. Goldman HJ, Littman ML, Oppenheimer GD, et al. Monilial cystitis: effective treatment with instillation of amphotericin B. *JAMA* 1960;174:359–362.
20. Wise GJ, Kozinn PJ, Goldberg PE. Amphotericin B as a urologic irrigant in the management of noninvasive candiduria. *J Urol* 1982;128:82–84.
21. Fisher JF, Chew WH, Smith S, et al. Urinary tract infections due to Candida albicans. *Rev Infect Dis* 1982;4:1107–1118.
22. Odds FC. *Candida plus candidosis.* Baltimore: University Park Press; 1979:147–153.
23. Hills JT. Candidiasis of urinary tract. *Proc R Soc Med* 1974;67:1155–1156.
24. Robinson PJ, Pocock RD, Frank JD. The management of obstructive renal candidiasis in the neonate. *Br J Urol* 1967;59:380–382.
25. Galleli JF. Assay and stability of amphotericin B in aqueous solution. *Drug Intell* 1967;1:102–105.
26. Solomkin JS, Flohr AB, Quie PS. The role of Candida in intraperitoneal infection. *Surgery* 1980;88:524–530.
27. Rahko PS, Davey WP, Wheat LJ, et al. Treatment of Torulopsis glabrata peritonitis with intraperitoneal amphotericin B. *JAMA* 1983;249:1187–1188.

28. Bastani B, Westervelt FB Jr. Persistence of Candida despite seemingly adequate systemic and intraperitoneal amphotericin B treatment in a patient on CAPD. *Am J Kidney Dis* 1986;8:265–267.
29. Bangham AD. Liposomes: realizing their promise. *Hosp Prac* 1992;27:51–62.
30. Ringden O, Meunier F, Tollemar J, et al. Efficacy of amphotericin B encapsulated in liposomes (AmBisome) in the treatment of invasive fungal infection in immunocompromised patients. *J Antimicrob Chemother* 1991;73(Suppl B):82.
31. Ralph ED, Barber KR, Grant CW. Liposomal amphotericin B: an effective, nontoxic preparation for the treatment of urinary tract infection caused by Candida albicans. *Am J Nephrol* 1991;11:118–122.
32. Block ER, Bennett JE. Pharmacological studies with 5- fluorocytosine. *Antimicrob Agents Chemother* 1972;1:476–482.
33. Schoenebeck J. Fungal infections of the urinary tract. In: Walsh PC, et al., eds. *Campbell's urology.* 5th ed. Philadelphia: WB Saunders; 1986:1025–1035.
34. Harder EJ, Hermans PE. Treatment of fungal infections with flucytosine. *Arch Intern Med* 1975;135:231–237.
35. Wise GJ, Kozinn PJ, Goldberg P. Flucytosine in the management of genitourinary candidiasis: 5 years' experience. *J Urol* 1980;124:70–72.
36. Meyer R, Axelrod JL. Fatal aplastic anemia resulting from flucytosine. *JAMA* 1974;228:1573.
37. Schoenebeck J, Segebrand E. Candida albicans septicaemia during first half of pregnancy successfully treated with 5-fluorocytosine. *Br Med J* 1973;4:337–338.
38. Schoenebeck J, Steen L, Tarnvick A. 5-Fluorocytosine treatment of Candida infections of the urinary tract and other sites. *Scand J Nephrol Urol* 1972;6:37–38.
39. Isacson M, Noah Z, Faber J, et al. Use of 5-fluorocytosine in systemic candidiasis in infancy. *Arch Dis Child* 1972;47:954–959.
40. Vandevelde AG, Mauceri AR, Johnson JE. 5-Fluorocytosine in the treatment of mycotic infections. *Ann Intern Med* 1972;77:43–52.
41. Bloch B, Kretzel A. Econazole nitrate in the treatment of candidal vaginitis. *S Afr Med J* 1980;58:314–316.
42. Wise GJ, Goldberg PE, Kozinn PJ. Do the imidazoles have role in the management of genitourinary fungal infections. *J Urol* 1985;133:61–64.
43. Wise GJ, Goldman WM, Goldberg PE, et al. Miconazole: a cost effective antifungal genitourinary irrigant. *J Urol* 1987;138:1413–1415.
44. Douhet E, Dupont B. Laboratory and clinical assessment of ketoconazole in deep-seated mycoses. Am J Med 1983;74(Suppl 1B):30–47.
45. Trachtenberg J, Halpern N, Pont A. Ketoconazole: a novel and rapid treatment for advanced prostatic cancer. *J Urol* 1983;130:152–153.
46. Bardare M, Tororano AM, Pietrogrande MC, et al. Pharmacokinetics of ketoconazole and treatment evaluation in candidal infections. *Arch Dis Child* 1984;59:1068–1071.
47. Saule H. Treatment of severe Candida infections with ketoconazole in newborn and young infants. *Dtsch Med Wochenschr* 1983;108:1676–1680.
48. Trenk D, Brett W, Jahnsen E, et al. Time course of cyclosporin/itraconazole interaction. *Lancet* 1987;2:1335–1338.
49. Bailey EM, Krakovsky DJ, Rybak MJ. The triazole antifungal agents: a review of itraconazole and fluconazole. *Pharmacotherapy* 1990;10 (2):146–153.
50. Brammer KW, Farrow PR, Faulkner JK. Pharmakcokinetics tissue penetration of fluconazole in humans. *Rev Infect Dis* 1990;12:S318–S326.
51. Lazer JD, Hilligoss DM. The clinical pharmacology of fluconazole. *Semin Oncol* 1990;17:14–18.
52. Anaissie E, Bodey GP, Kantarjian H. Fluconazole therapy for chronic disseminated candidiasis in patient with leukemia and prior amphotericin B therapy. *Am J Med* 1991;91:142–150.
53. Viscoli C, Castagnola E, Fioredda F, et al. Fluconazole in the treatment of candidiasis in immunocompromised children. *Antimicrob Agents Chemother* 1991;35:365–367.
54. Bodey GP. Azole antifungal Agents. *Clin Infect Dis* 1992;14(Suppl 1):S161–S169.
55. Tucker RM, Denning DW, Dupont B, Stevens DA. Itraconazole therapy for chronic coccidioidal meningitis. *Ann Intern Med* 1990;112:108–112.

56. Itraconazole. *Med Lett Drugs Ther* 1993;35:7.
57. Moreno F, Hardin TC, Rinaldi MG, Graybill JR. Itraconazole-didanosine excipient interaction. *JAMA* 1993;269:1508.
58. Viviani AM, Tortorano, AM, Pagano A, et al. European experience with itraconazole in systemic mycoses. *J Am Acad Dermatol* 1990;23(3, Part 2):587–593.
59. Schulkind ML, Ayoub GM. Transfer factor and its clinical application. *Adv Pediatr* 1980;27:89–116.
60. Petranyi G, Ryder NS, Stutz A. Allylamine derivatives: new class of synthetic antifungal agents inhibiting fungal squalene expoxidase. *Science* 1984;224:1239–1241.
61. Grunberg RN, Leakey A. Treatment of candidal urinary tract infection with nifuratel. *Br Med J* 1976;2:908–910.
62. Bacigalupo A, Van Lint MT, Fraibboni F, et al. Mepartricin: a new antifungal agent for the treatment of disseminated Candida infections in the immunocompromised host. *Acta Haematol* 1983;69:409–413.
63. Krieger JN. Vaginitis: current concepts of etiology, diagnosis and treatment. *AUA Update Series* 1983;35(part 1):1–5.
64. Wallenburg HC, Wladimiroff JW. Recurrence of vulvovaginal candidosis during pregnancy: comparison of miconazole vs. nystatin treatment.*Obstet Gynecol* 1976;48:491–494.
65. Hann I, et al. Ketoconazole vs. nystatin plus amphotericin B for fungal prophylaxis in severely immunocompromised patients. *Lancet* 1982;1:826–829.
66. Stevens DA. Thrush can be prevented in patients with acquired immunodeficiency syndrome and the acquired immunodeficiency syndrome-related complex: randomized, double-blind, placebo-controlled study of 100-mg oral fluconazole daily. *Arch Intern Med* 1991;151:2458–2464.
67. Como JA, Dismukes WE. Oral azole drugs as systemic antifungal therapy. *New Engl J Med* 1994;330:263–272.

Antibiotic Therapy in Urology,
edited by S. Grant Mulholland, M.D.,
Lippincott-Raven Publishers, Philadelphia © 1996.

Chapter 9

Problems Associated with Outpatient Antibiotic Usage

Robert M. Moldwin and *Joseph Del Pizzo

*Albert Einstein College of Medicine, Department of Urology, Long Island Jewish Medical Center, New Hyde Park, New York 11042; *Department of Urology, University of Maryland, Baltimore, Maryland 21201*

It was August in Southern California. Dr. Mather was treating Mr. Smith for chronic bacterial prostatitis with a 6-week course of fluoroquinolone therapy. One week later, Mr. Smith presented to Dr. Mather with second-degree burns over his face, chest, and legs. Dr. Mather unfortunately forgot to inform the patient about potential phototoxicity with the use of fluoroquinolones and later found out that the patient was a lifeguard!

Ms. Able was treated by Dr. Wilkins for 3 months with antibiotic prophylaxis for recurrent episodes of bacterial cystitis using nitrofurantoin 100 mg qhs. Ms. Able was free from further episodes of cystitis; however, she reported to Dr. Wilkins that she felt a bit "under the weather" and had developed an annoying dry cough. Dr. Wilkins told Ms. Able that she might be catching the flu. Two weeks later, Ms. Able was seen in her local emergency room with shortness of breath. A chest x-ray revealed pulmonary fibrosis, one of the uncommon, often insidious, complications of nitrofurantoin therapy.

Outpatient therapy of uncomplicated and complicated urinary tract infections is usually successful and uneventful. However, as seen in the above illustrations, antibiotic administration can be the cause of significant morbidity. In most cases, complications associated with antibiotic therapy are the result of idiosyncratic reactions. Other complications are secondary to preventable drug-drug interactions or inappropriate antibiotic administration to a particular patient (1–5). Detailed knowledge of an antibiotic's safety profile is, therefore, as important as knowledge of its spectrum of activity and tissue penetration. This chapter reviews the classes of oral antibiotics frequently dispensed for the outpatient treatment of urinary tract infections and the potential problems associated with their use.

FLUOROQUINOLONES

Fluoroquinolones have had a major impact on the treatment of genitourinary infections because of their safety and wide spectrum of gram-negative (and to some extent gram-positive) coverage (6–10). Although not significantly more effective than other, less expensive, drugs in treating uncomplicated urinary tract infections, their high tissue penetration gives the quinolones a distinct clinical advantage in combatting complicated infections (11–13).

Adverse Effects

Halkin (14) reports that fluoroquinolones have an adverse reaction rate ranging from 4–8%. The adverse reaction profile is similar for all members of the fluoroquinolone group and necessitates discontinuation of therapy in only 1–2.6% of patients. Gastrointestinal symptoms are reported most often (3–6%), which include nausea, vomiting, abdominal discomfort, and diarrhea. Pseudomembranous colitis associated with *Clostridium difficile* is uncommon.

Central nervous system effects (1–4%) manifest as headaches, dizziness, agitation, sleep disturbances, and hallucinations (14). Although seen with all the fluoroquinolones, CNS reactions are more frequently noted with lomefloxacin. Seizures have been reported in patients with underlying CNS disturbances and are more likely to occur with the concurrent use of fluoroquinolones and nonsteroidal anti-inflammatory agents. The fluoroquinolones are, therefore, relatively contraindicated in patients with known seizure disorders or cerebrovascular disease (10). Cartilaginous erosions in diarthrodial weight-bearing joints are seen following prolonged quinolone dosing in immature mammals. Thus, these antibiotics are contraindicated in patients under 18 years of age, pregnant women, and nursing mothers.

Rare cases of interstitial nephritis, hematuria, and acute renal failure have been reported (10,14,15). Since the excretion of most fluoroquinolones is predominantly renal, renal failure may necessitate dosage reduction. Norfloxacin and ciprofloxacin have significant hepatic excretion, and dosage reduction is required only for a creatinine clearance of less than 30 ml/min. In very high doses, crystalluria may occur in patients with alkaline urine, but it has not been associated with renal toxicity or calculus formation.

Although skin reactions such as rash or pruritus appear infrequently (0.5–2.0%), photosensitivity is often reported. Moderate-to-severe phototoxicity reactions have been observed in patients exposed to direct sunlight while receiving fluoroquinolone therapy. All patients should be advised to avoid excessive sunlight while receiving these antibiotics and to discontinue therapy if phototoxicity occurs.

Drug Interactions

Numerous drug interactions with the fluoroquinolones have been established (16,17). Several of these antibiotics significantly interact with methylxanthine compounds and may promote serious or fatal reactions (Table 1). Enoxacin and ciprofloxacin are known to decrease the total body clearance of theophylline through inhibition of the hepatic catabolism of theophylline. Davies and Maesen (17) showed that enoxacin brought about a reduction of total body theophylline clearance of 64%; ciprofloxacin decreased clearance by 30%. These drug interactions require close monitoring of theophylline levels if concurrent dosing is performed. Symptoms of accumulation of the methylxanthines include agitation, restlessness, and nausea. Ofloxacin, norfloxacin, and lomefloxacin do not demonstrate clinically significant interactions with methylxanthines. Quinolones have also been demonstrated to interact with the methylxanthine caffeine. The most significant effects (agitation, tremor, confusion) are seen with enoxacin, with which a 78% reduction in caffeine clearance was found (17). A less significant effect was seen with ciprofloxacin. Patients should, therefore, be advised to limit caffeine intake during quinolone therapy.

Sodium warfarin and related drugs are hepatically metabolized via the same pathway as theophylline. Thus, administration of sodium warfarin and a fluoroquinolone mandates close monitoring of prothrombin time.

Absorption of all of the fluoroquinolones from the upper gastrointestinal tract is greatly reduced by binding to antacids containing magnesium, calcium, or aluminum salts and to iron or zinc dietary supple-

TABLE 1. *Interaction between quinolone antibiotics, methylxanthines, and antacids*

Quinolone	Interference with xanthine elimination		Effect of antacids on absorption
	Theophylline	Caffeine	
Ciprofloxacin	+ to +++	++	+++
Enoxacin	+++	+++	++
Lomefloxacin	no effect	no effect	++
Norfloxacin	+	no effect	+++
Ofloxacin	+ to no effect	no effect	++
Pefloxacin	+		++

From Davies and Maesen, ref. 17.

ments (16). Likewise, sucralfate may bind to the fluoroquinolones, leading to decreased antibiotic absorption. Patients should be advised not take these binding medications up to 4 hours before or within 2 hours after taking the antibiotic. Milk products do not significantly interact with the quinolone antibiotics.

Probenecid, which blocks renal tubular secretion, increases serum levels of those fluoroquinolones with primarily renal excretion (i.e., pefloxacin, 60%; ofloxacin, 80%). Cimetidine, a commonly prescribed H_2 blocker, may interfere with the elimination of the fluoroquinolones; such an interaction has been demonstrated with pefloxacin (17,18).

Bacterial Resistance

The emergence of organisms resistant to the fluoroquinolones is relatively uncommon, being seen in fewer than 2% of patients treated for uncomplicated urinary tract infection (19). Fluoroquinolones produce their effects by inhibition of bacterial DNA gyrase, an enzyme responsible for the supercoiling of bacterial DNA and for bacterial DNA repair mechanisms. Resistance to the fluoroquinolones appears to be mediated by a spontaneous point mutation that results in an altered DNA gyrase enzyme and occurs at a frequency of less than 1 in 10^{10} bacteria. Other reported mechanisms of resistance include changes in bacterial cell membrane permeability (seen with *Escherichia coli* and *Pseudomonas aeruginosa*) and the development of cell membrane-based efflux pumps (seen with *Staphylococcus aureus* and *E. coli*). The bacterial acquisition of resistance to one fluoroquinolone usually confers resistance to other fluoroquinolones and, in some cases, to structurally unrelated drugs such as β-lactam antibiotics, tetracycline, and chloramphenicol. The emergence of resistance is commonly seen with *P. aeruginosa* and *S. aureus*. In the case of *Pseudomonas*, the frequency of the single-step mutation to quinolone resistance is 1000-fold more common than in *E. coli* (20).

Indiscriminate use of the fluoroquinolones appears to be a key factor in the acquisition of resistance. In Spain, where these antibiotics can be purchased "over the counter," the resistance rate of community-acquired *E. coli* infections climbed from less than 1% to 8.1% in 3 years (21)!

URINARY ANTISEPTICS

The urinary tract antiseptics are a varied group of agents that achieve high urinary concentrations, making them effective in treating acute uncomplicated urinary tract infections.

The major drugs placed in this class include nitrofurantoin, nalidixic acid, and methenamine.

Nitrofurantoin

Nitrofurantoin is primarily excreted unchanged in the urine, achieving high urinary concentrations against *E. coli*, *S. saprophyticus*, and enterococci. Although detected in renal interstitial tissue, nitrofurantoin achieves very low concentrations in serum or other tissues.

Nitrofurantoin is not found in vaginal secretions. Hence, vaginal flora is unchanged and therapy is not associated with yeast vaginitis (22,23). Nitrofurantoin's low tissue penetration makes it a poor choice for invasive tissue infections (i.e., acute bacterial prostatitis, pyelonephritis).

Adverse Effects

The most common adverse reactions involve the gastrointestinal tract, where the incidence is reported at 5–7%. Reactions include nausea, vomiting, and diarrhea (24). These problems can be circumvented by reduction in dosage, concurrent intake of food, and the use of macrocystalline forms (Macrobid, Macrodantin). Skin rashes are the next most common reaction, occurring in 1% of patients.

A variety of hematologic reactions have been reported, including hemolytic anemia in individuals who are deficient in glucose-6-phosphate dehydrogenase (G-6-PD). Although nitrofurantoin may be dispensed during pregnancy, it is contraindicated in patients with a family history of this genetic disorder. These abnormalities are usually reversible following withdrawal of the drug (24).

Reversible and irreversible peripheral polyneuropathy has been reported and is more likely to arise in patients with diabetes mellitus, anemia, or moderate renal insufficiency.

The most feared complications of nitrofurantoin therapy are pulmonary hypersensitivity reactions. Patients may present with acute pulmonary edema, chest pain, and a peripheral eosinophilia. Malaise, a chronic dry cough, or shortness of breath may be symptoms of interstitial fibrosis or interstitial pneumonitis. In such cases, nitrofurantoin therapy should be stopped immediately. The patient should then be evaluated with a chest x-ray and, if warranted, pulmonary function testing. Pulmonary function may be permanently altered. The best chance for recovery of pulmonary function rests with rapid diagnosis and drug cessation (25).

Resistance

Nitrofurantoin's antibacterial activity is thought to be based on its (or its metabolic intermediate's) nonspecific binding to bacterial ribosomal proteins, resulting in broad-based inhibition of protein synthesis. This mechanism may explain the historically low bacterial resistance rate to this drug. Recently, however, bacterial resistance to nitrofurantoin by organisms commonly associated with uncomplicated cystitis has been reported and ranges from 15–20% (26). The mechanism of resistance is presently unknown.

Drug Interactions

Magnesium salts have been shown to decrease nitrofurantoin absorption and result in inadequate drug concentrations in the urine. Nitrofurantoin should be taken with meals since food appears to minimize the antibiotic's gastrointestinal side effects and may increase its bioavailability by 40% (27).

Nalidixic Acid

The use of nalidixic acid (NegGram) in the urologic setting has decreased since the introduction of its systemically acting congeners, the quinolones. Ten percent to 15% of nalidixic acid is found in its antibacterial hydroxylated form, hydroxynalidixic acid. This urinary antiseptic nonetheless has good antimicrobial activity against the common uropathogens that cause uncomplicated urinary tract infection (28).

Adverse Effects

As with nitrofurantoin, the most commonly reported side effects of nalidixic acid are gastrointestinal. Hypersensitivity reactions are also seen, the most prevalent being photosensitivity reactions (28). Nalidixic acid should not be given to infants or patients with pre-existing cerebrovascular symptomatology since reversible neurologic side effects (headache, dizziness, confusion, and malaise) are more commonly reported (29,30).

Rarely, nalidixic acid has resulted in hepatic injury characterized by liver function study abnormalities and jaundice. Hemolytic anemia has been reported in patients with G-6-PD deficiency. Physicians prescribing dosing for longer than 2 weeks should monitor liver function and blood counts (31).

Drug Interactions

Nalidixic acid is known to enhance the effects of oral anticoagulants, such as warfarin, by displacing significant amounts from serum albumin binding sites. Significant bleeding episodes may occur in patients receiving both drugs (16).

Resistance

The emergence of bacterial resistance can be a problem, particularly in *E. coli* infections, with rates of bacterial resistance ranging from 6–26% (30). In the laboratory, bacterial resistance to naladixic acid occurs 6 to 7 orders of magnitude more frequently than to the fluoroquinolones (19). If bacterial resistance to nalidixic acid emerges during treatment, it usually does so within the first 48 hours, permitting rapid change to another antimicrobial regimen. Underdosage with nalidixic acid during initial therapy using less than 4g/day for adults may facilitate bacterial resistance (30).

Methenamine

Methenamine is frequently used in combination with hippurate (methenamine hippurate, Hiprex) and with mandelate (methenamine mandelate, Mandelamine) for acute infections and as prophylaxis for recurrent infections in children and adults. The methenamine component is hydrolyzed in acidic urine (pH <6.0) to formaldehyde, thereby providing antiseptic activity. Hippurate and mandelate serve to keep the urine acidic in addition to possessing some antimicrobial activity of their own. Care must therefore be taken to maintain an acid pH of the urine, especially when treating infections caused by urea-splitting organisms such as *Proteus* and strains of *Pseudomonas*. These agents are effective only in urine and are contraindicated for the treatment of invasive infections.

Adverse Effects

Methenamine and its acid salts are very well tolerated and rarely induce systemic toxicity. Minor adverse reactions include nausea, gastric irritation, dysuria, and rash. The overall incidence of reactions is reported as 1–7% (32). These symptoms are believed to be secondary to the local effects of formaldehyde (33). Higher doses or prolonged administration of methenamine (>8.0g/day for 3 to 4 weeks) have resulted in bladder irritation, painful and frequent micturition, albuminuria, and gross hematuria.

Acid salts should not be prescribed to patients with renal insufficiency or gout because they can cause crystalluria. Methenamine base is readily converted to formaldehyde and is not a problem in azotemic patients. Methenamine and sulfonamides should not be administered concurrently since formaldehyde and sulfonamides form insoluble precipitates. Thiazide diuretics, carbonic anhydrase inhibitors, antacids, or urinary alkalinizing agents should not be administered with methenamine since they inhibit the drug's conversion to formaldehyde (33).

PENICILLINS

The preferred groups of penicillins for the treatment of uncomplicated urinary tract infections are the aminopenicillins (i.e., ampicillin, amoxicillin) and combinations of aminopenicillins and β-lactamase inhibitors. These agents are superior to penicillin in terms of their spectrum of microbial coverage and lower bacterial resistance rates. The advantage of the carboxypenicillins and the ureidopenicillins are their enhanced anti-Pseudomonal activity. They therefore play a more important role in the treatment of nosocomial infections than in community-acquired infections of the urinary tract.

Aminopenicillins

The aminopenicillins were the first group of penicillins to act against gram-negative bacteria. As a result, ampicillin and amoxicillin became long-standing favorites for the treatment of urinary tract infections. More recently, these agents have been relegated to second- or third-line therapy because of increasing bacterial resistance and significantly greater treatment failure rates compared with sulfonamides and quinolones (34–36).

Adverse Effects

The adverse effects of ampicillin and amoxicillin are similar. Use of these antibiotics is often associated with the development of yeast vaginitis (14–25%) since they often eradicate normal vaginal flora, potentiating monilial overgrowth (37). This problem has been partially circumvented in the treatment of uncomplicated bacterial cystitis with shorter courses of therapy (3-day therapy rather than therapy for 7 to 10 days).

Hypersensitivity reactions are the next most common complaints, occurring in approximately 8% of patients and ranging from skin rashes to immediate anaphylaxis. Anaphylactic reactions are rare, occurring in fewer than 0.2% of cases and having a 0.001% mortality. Late skin reactions (rashes) are seen more commonly with aminopenicillins than with any other class of penicillins. Early skin reactions (urticaria) are more prevalent with penicillin G and are not associated with ampicillin or amoxicillin.

Ampicillin is poorly absorbed from the gastrointestinal tract. The fecal concentration is often three times as high as the urinary levels. Enteric flora may be altered, thereby causing abdominal pain, nausea, and diarrhea. Amoxicillin is better absorbed through the gastrointestinal tract, and therefore diarrhea is a less common complaint. In addition, long courses of penicillin therapy can induce pseudomembranous colitis secondary to *Clostridium difficile* superinfection.

Ampicillin may cause interstitial nephritis in patients taking large doses over an extended period of time. Potential bleeding complications associated with the use of β-lactam antibiotics leading to immune destruction of erythrocytes, leukocytes, and platelets are extremely rare and usually reversible on withdrawal of the drug (38).

Drug Interactions

Reported pharmacologic drug interactions involving the aminopenicillins are limited to ampicillin. The incidence of allergic skin rash associated with ampicillin is three times higher during use of allopurinol (16).

Dossetor and colleagues (39) reported three cases of women on oral contraception who became pregnant while taking ampicillin. They attributed the contraceptive failure to an interaction between the two medications. The risk of oral contraceptive failure with concomitant ampicillin use is unpredictable yet potentially devastating to the patient. Patients should be advised to use an alternative method of contraception during antibiotic treatment.

Bacterial Resistance

The mechanisms of resistance to β-lactam antibiotics through alteration of penicillin-binding proteins, cell wall permeability changes, and production of β-lactamases are well known. Of these mechanisms, hydrolysis of the β-lactam ring accounts for the majority of organisms with resistance to amoxicillin and ampicillin. Rates of microbial resistance to these antibiotics have been reported as high as 35% in the treatment of acute uncomplicated urinary tract infections and have led to the use of β-lactamase inhibitors to circumvent this problem (36).

Penicillins plus β-Lactamase Inhibitors

The two currently available β-lactamase inhibitors are clavulanic acid and sulbactam. These agents have high affinity and irreversible binding to bacterial β-lactamases, thereby preventing the hydrolysis of the antibiotic's β-lactam ring. In addition, β-lactamase inhibitors have weak antibacterial activity, which has an additive effect when they are used in conjunction with a penicillin. Available agents include clavulanic acid (amoxicillin plus clavulanic acid, Augmentin) and sulbactam (ampicillin plus sulbactam, Unasyn). These antimicrobials are useful against most β-lactamase-producing strains of *E. coli*, *S. aureus*, *S. epidermidis*, *Klebsiella*, and *Proteus*, and they are commonly used to treat uncomplicated infections of the lower urinary tract. They are also used in parenteral form to treat more serious infections of the urinary tract.

Adverse Effects

These combination agents retain the safety of the original β-lactam component; however, the adverse effects are also retained. Yeast vaginitis is still very much a problem. The gastrointestinal side effects seen with both groups of penicillins are rarely severe enough to interfere with patient compliance and can be alleviated by dosing after meals.

Resistance

Both clavulanic acid and sulbactam are effective at inhibiting β-lactamases in Richmond-Sykes classes II through V but not in class I. Clavulanic acid has been reported to induce class I β-lactamase production (40). Augmentin (amoxicillin plus clavulanic acid) also appears to predispose patients to reinfection with ampicillin-resistant strains.

CEPHALOSPORINS

The three generations of cephalosporin antibiotics offer broad-spectrum bactericidal activity. The first- and second-generation cephalosporins are active against almost all gram-positive bacteria as well as against most common aerobic gram-negative enterics, such as *E. coli*, *Klebsiella*, and *Proteus* species. Third-generation antibiotics have less activity against gram-positive organisms but extend gram-negative coverage to include stains of *P. aeruginosa*, *Serratia*, and *Citrobacter*. Their use as first-line treatment for uncomplicated urinary tract infections is limited by their relatively high cost and negligible clinical advantage over less expensive, equally efficacious alternative antibiotics.

Adverse Effects

As a group, cephalosporins have a favorable profile of toxicity. Hypersensitivity or allergic reactions are most common. Rash, pruritus, and urticaria occur in approximately 1–3% of patients and are most commonly reported with cefoperazone (Cefobid) and ceftriaxone (Rocephin) (41,42). Patients with a history of penicillin allergy are more likely to develop these problems (incidence, 5.4–16.5%) than patients with no penicillin allergy (incidence, 0.5–1.2%). Severe hypersensitivity/anaphylaxis is rare.

Cephalosporins are a common cause of drug fever, this being reported in 5–15% of patients receiving greater than 10 days of therapy. Hematologic abnormalities are rare and are related to the parenterally administered agents with a methylthiotetrazole (MTT) side chain, such as cefoperazone, cefmetazole, and moxalactam. The MTT side chain impairs synthesis of vitamin K-dependent clotting factors. This may be blocked prophylactically by administering vitamin K during cephalosporin therapy. Other infrequent adverse effects include diarrhea, thrombophlebitis, and clinical superinfection with species of *Candida.*

Drug Interactions

Those cephalosporins containing an MTT side chain may inhibit acetaldehyde metabolism and cause a disulfiram-type reaction when taken with alcohol (43). They should be administered with caution to patients taking warfarin or heparin because of their interaction with vitamin K-dependent clotting factors (16).

Bacterial Resistance

Bacterial resistance to cephalosporins, as with the penicillins, is primarily based on chromosomal or plasmid-mediated β-lactamase activity. Other mechanisms of acquired resistance may include cell wall permeability changes and altered binding to intracytoplasmic protein receptors. Most gram-negative aerobic microorganisms have chromosomal β-lactamases that may be induced by environmental agents. First-generation cephalosporins and cefoxitin are strong inducers of these β-lactamases. The remainder of the second- and third-generation agents are weak inducers. Those organisms with inducible β-lactamases include species of *Enterobacter*, *Serratia*, *Citrobacter*, *Morganella*, *Providencia*, *Proteus*, and *Pseudomonas*. The rapid development of antibiotic resistance for such organisms ranges between 14% and 56% (42). Unfortunately, in vitro antibiotic sensitivity testing is unreliable in this setting (falsely indicating bacterial sensitivity) and may lead to therapeutic failures.

TRIMETHOPRIM/SULFAMETHOXAZOLE

Trimethoprim plus sulfamethoxazole (TMP/SMX) has gained prominence in both the short-course treatment and prophylaxis of lower urinary tract infections (44–48). In combination, these drugs inhibit two steps in folate metabolism. (Folate is needed by many bacteria for nucleic acid synthesis, while mammalian cells depend upon exogenous sources.) Sulfonamides are competitive inhibitors of the bacterial enzyme responsible for the conversion of *p*-aminobenzoate to dihydropteroic acid, the immediate precursor to folic acid. Trimethoprim competitively inhibits the activity of bacterial dihydrofolate reductase. This enzyme reduces dihydrofolic to tetrahydrofolic acid, a step in the synthesis of purines and ultimately bacterial DNA. Trimethoprim inhibits bacterial dihydrofolate reductase 50,000 times more efficiently than in mammalian cells. The combination of TMP/SMX produces a synergistic bactericidal effect against many gram-positive and gram-negative bacteria (44,49,50).

Adverse Effects

The incidence of serious adverse reactions associated with the use of TMP/SMX is low. Jick (51) reported incidences of anaphylaxis, superinfection, and hematologic effects such as agranulocytosis, thrombocytopenia, leukopenia, and hemolytic anemia as less than 1% (51). TMP/SMX should be used with caution in patients with suspected folate deficiency (i.e., chronic alcoholics, malnourished patients, elderly). Like nitrofurantoin, sulfonamides may cause hemolysis in patients with G-6-PD deficiency. Long-term use of TMP/SMX should be monitored with complete blood counts.

Sulfonamides pass placental barriers and are found in breast milk. They displace bilirubin from plasma-binding proteins and may cause neonatal jaundice and kernicterus. Sulfonamides are, therefore, contraindicated in nursing mothers and in the third trimester of pregnancy. Severe cutaneous skin eruptions, including Stevens-Johnson syndrome, have been reported with sulfonamide administration, but the frequency of its occurrence is also rare (<1%) (52,53). The medication should be discontinued at the first sign of rash. More frequent but less serious side effects include nausea and vomiting (3.2%), diarrhea (1.5%), and cutaneous allergic and mild cutaneous hypersensitivity reactions (3.4%).

Side effects are often dose-related. A randomized comparison of single doses, and 3-day and 10-day courses of TMP/SMX in 300 women revealed that the incidence of adverse reactions was significantly greater in patients treated with the 10-day course (28%) than in those treated with the 3-day course (9%) or a single dose (3%) (54,55). In regard to prophylaxis, Labbe (56) demonstrated an 11% incidence of side effects in patients receiving daily prophylaxis and a 3% incidence in patients when prophylaxis was limited to three times per week (56).

It has been well established that patients with acquired immune deficiency syndrome (AIDS) have a much higher incidence of exaggerated adverse reactions to TMP/SMX (57,58). Jick (51) reports a frequency of adverse reactions as high as 70%, especially serious skin reactions, cytopenias, and hepatotoxicity.

Early studies demonstrated that sulfonamides of low solubility readily crystallized in the renal parenchyma and urinary tracts (59). This crystallization might lead to oliguric renal failure and allergic and hypersensitivity reactions resembling allergic interstitial nephritis and obstructive nephropathy. Fortunately, crystalline nephropathy has become relatively rare (0.2–0.4%) with the introduction of short-acting sulfonamides of equal potency but greater solubility, such as sulfamethoxazole and sulfisoxazole (59). Crystalluria, however, may still become a problem when using higher doses of TMP/SMX, particularly in dehydrated patients with pre-xisting renal disease.

Drug Interactions

Several significant drug interactions occur with the sulfonamides. TMP/SMX may enhance the effects of warfarin and sulfonylureas by displacing these drugs from plasma proteins and through impairment of their metabolism by the liver. Physicians should avoid concomitant use of these drugs, as bleeding episodes and hypoglycemia have been reported (16). The use of TMP/SMX with phenytoin may lead to toxic serum phenytoin levels. Serum phenytoin concentrations should be closely monitored during sulfonamide treatment.

Bacterial Resistance

Treatment failure with the sulfonamides results most commonly from the emergence of TMP/SMX-resistant strains among *E. coli* and *Klebsiella* species. The development of resistant organisms is both chromosome- and/or plasmid-mediated and is high for both trimethoprim and sulfamethoxazole when they are used as single agents. Antibiotic resistance is lower when they are given in combination (50); however, resistance of organisms associated with uncomplicated bacterial cystitis now varies from 5–15% in the United States to 25% in Western Europe (21).

TRIMETHOPRIM

Trimethoprim (Proloprim) as a single agent is used for the initial treatment of uncomplicated urinary tract infections caused by susceptible strains of *E. coli*, *Klebsiella pneumoniae*, *Proteus*, *Enterobacter*, and coagulase-negative *Staphylococcus* species. Like TMP/SMX, it should be given with caution to patients with possible folate deficiency and those taking phenytoin. The adverse effect profile is similar to the TMP/SMX combination, with rash, pruritus, and phototoxic skin eruptions being the most commonly encountered problems.

TETRACYCLINES

As a group, the tetracyclines are now used less frequently to treat urinary tract infections, in large part because of the development of antimicrobial resistance among uropathogens and the appearance of newer, more effective agents. The tetracyclines continue to play a role in the management of urologic infections on the basis of their high urinary concentration and their value in the treatment of *Chlamydia* and *Ureaplasma* infections (60–62).

Adverse Effects

Gastrointestinal irritation is a frequent side effect, especially with the use of oxytetracycline and doxycycline hyclate. Tetracyclines are very acidic in solution, and esophageal ulcerations occurring in patients with pre-existing gastroesophageal disease are occasionally seen (60,62). Such patients should be encouraged to take these drugs with liberal amounts of fluid (not milk or other dairy products) or antacids (those not containing aluminum, magnesium, or calcium).

Superinfections, especially oral and anogenital candidiasis, are common in patients taking a tetracycline. Vaginal candidiasis occurs in up to 25% of women receiving tetracycline therapy (62). Diarrhea may occur because of superinfection with *Staphylococcus* or, less frequently, colonization with *Clostridium difficile*.

Photosensitivity is a classic toxic reaction, most commonly seen with doxycycline and demeclocycline.

Tetracyclines cause brown discoloration of the teeth and may retard growth of bone in the human fetus and children. Doxycycline is less likely than the other tetracyclines to cause this reaction. These medications should not be administered to pregnant women, nursing mothers, or children under 12 years of age. Administration to pregnant women is also contraindicated because fatal reactions caused by hepatotoxicity have been reported (62).

Tetracyclines are known to increase the occurrence of azotemia by drug-induced reduction of protein synthesis, resulting in protein metabolism. They should be used with extreme caution or avoided in patients with pre-existing renal disease. Doxycycline is safer as it has enhanced gastrointestinal absorption.

There are reports of drug-related vestibular toxicity manifested by dizziness, ataxia, and vomiting with minocycline therapy (62). Patients should be informed to discontinue use of the antibiotic should these signs of neurotoxicity occur.

Drug Interactions

Divalent metals (calcium, magnesium, and aluminum) form chelates with all tetracyclines, inhibiting the gastrointestinal absorption of the antibiotics. Antacids containing these metals should be avoided during tetracycline therapy. If antacids must be used, the patient should be informed to take tetracycline doses 2 to 3 hours before or after the antacid dose. Substitution of an H_2 antagonist for the antacid should be considered. Doxycycline has decreased calcium binding and may be taken with milk products but not with antacids.

Anticonvulsants increase the hepatic catabolism of doxycycline and compromise the antimicrobial efficacy of the drug. Substitution of tetracycline for doxycycline is effective since the former exerts minimal effect on hepatic enzymes.

Renal failure has been reported in patients receiving tetracycline therapy after general anesthesia with methoxyflurane (63). The renal failure was secondary to formation of calcium oxalate crystals. Renal problems may also occur when tetracyclines are administered concomitantly with diuretics. Patients should, therefore, be well hydrated prior to tetracycline therapy.

As seen with ampicillin, tetracycline may decrease the efficacy of oral birth control medications. Patients should be advised of this potential problem and potentially select alternative methods of birth control.

Bacterial Resistance

Resistance to the tetracyclines appears slowly, is incremental, and has been reported to occur in up to 21% of patients receiving the drug to treat uncomplicated cystitis (64). Resistance is imparted by plasmids that encode proteins responsible for disabling active transport of the drug through the inner cytoplasmic membrane. Development of resistance necessitates institution of a different class of antibiotic, as microorganisms that acquire resistance to one tetracycline are usually resistant to the other members of that class.

MONOBACTAMS

This relatively new group of antibiotics has a directed spectrum of activity, similar to that of the aminoglycosides, against gram-negative aerobic bacteria. Aztreonam is a useful urologic antibiotic because of its activity against many uropathogens, including strains of *Pseudomonas*, *Serratia*, *E. coli*, *Klebsiella*, *Enterobacter*, and *Citrobacter*, and it can be used as single-dose therapy to treat uncomplicated cystitis (65–67).

Adverse Effects

Madsen et al. (68) reported a low incidence of adverse experiences in aztreonam-treated patients with urinary tract infection. In patients receiving a single dose for uncomplicated cystitis, the prevalence of side effects was 1.7%, whereas in those cases in which multiple doses were needed to eradicate a complicated infection, adverse effects were seen in 6.8% of cases. Discontinuation of therapy was necessary in 2% of cases.

The most frequently reported adverse effects included rash (2%), phlebitis (2%), and diarrhea (1%) (69). Madsen et al. reported a 5% prevalence of superinfection, most commonly with group D streptococci and staphylococci (68).

Bacterial Resistance

Aztreonam is unique among β-lactam compounds in that it shows a high degree of stability to β-lactamase, imparting significant activity against multiple antibiotic-resistant strains of gram-negative bacteria. Resistant strains of bacteria may emerge in 3–4% of cases through enzyme induction. Cross-resistance may occur between aztreonam and other β-lactam antibiotics (65).

CONCLUSIONS

Urinary tract infections account for 5.2 million office visits per year and lead to approximately 100,000 hospitalizations (70). Untoward reactions to antimicrobial therapy are usually quite low; however, the high numbers of patients requiring treatment suggest that physicians often encounter these problems in practice. Many reactions are completely unpredictable, but careful attention to the patient's past medical history can frequently circumvent disasters in patient care.

REFERENCES

1. Parsons CL. Protocol for treatment of typical urinary tract infection: criteria for antimicrobial selection. *Urology* 1988;32(Suppl):2.
2. Hanno PM. Therapeutic principles of antimicrobial therapy and new antimicrobial agents. *Urol Clin North Am* 1986;13:4.
3. Elder NC. Acute urinary tract infection in women. *Postgrad Med* 1992;92:6.
4. Johnson JR. Urinary tract infection: selecting the optimal agent. *Drug Ther* 1991;1:27.
5. Goldstein EJC. Prevention of bacterial resistance in urinary tract infections. *Eur Urol* 1991;19(Suppl):235.
6. Hooper DC, Wolfson J. Fluoroquinolone antimicrobial agents. *New Engl J Med* 1991;324:1100.
7. Zinner SH. Clinical use of oral fluoroquinolone antibiotics. *Infect Med* 1993;10:43.
8. Naber KG. Use of quinolones in urinary tract infections and prostatitis. *Rev Infect Dis* 1989;11(Suppl 5):1321.
9. Dalkin BL, Schaeffer AJ. Fluoroquinolone antimicrobial agents. *Probl Urol* 1988;2:476.
10. Ball P. Long term use of quinolones and their safety. *Rev Infect Dis* 1989;11(Suppl 5): S1365–1370.
11. Hooper D, Wolfson J. Treatment of genitorurinary tract infections with fluoroquinolones: clinical efficacy in genital infections and adverse effects. *Antimicrob Agents Chemother* 1989;33:10.
12. Sabbaj T, Hoagland VL, Shih WJ. Multiclinic comparative study of norfloxacin and trimethroprim-sulfamethoxazole for treatment of urinary tract infections. *Antimicrob Agents Chemother* 1985;27:297.
13. Corrado M. Worldwide clinical experience with ofloxacin in urologic cases. *Urology* 1991;37(Suppl):3.
14. Halkin H. Adverse effects of the fluoroquinolones. *Rev Infect Dis* 1988;10(Suppl 1): S258–261.
15. Christ W, Lehnert T, Ulbrich B. Specific toxicologic aspects of the quinolones. *Rev Infect Dis* 1988;10(Suppl 1):S141.
16. Lee M, Sharifi R. Avoiding antibiotic drug interactions. *Infect Urol* 1990;61:160.
17. Davies B, Maesen F. Drug interactions with quinolones. *Rev Infect Dis* 1989;11(Suppl 5): S1083–1090.
18. Sondheimer J. Toxic nephropathies in urologic infection. *Infect Urol* 1990;58:160.
19. Wolfson J, Hooper D. Bacterial resistance to quinolones: mechanisms and clinical importance. *Rev Infect Dis* 1989;11(Suppl 5):S960–968.
20. Hooper D, Wolfson J. Bacterial resistance to the quinolone antimicrobial agents. *Am J Med* 1989;87(Suppl 6C):120.
21. Ena J, Amador C, Martinez C, Ortiz de la Tabla V. Risk factors for aquisition of urinary tract infections caused by ciprofloxacin resistant Echerichia coli. *J Urol* 1995;153:117.
22. Dramer DL, Dodd MC. The mode of action of nitrofurantoin compounds. *J Bacteriol* 1946;51:293.

23. Schneider RE. Single-blind comparison of cinoxacin and nitrofurantoin in the treatment of urinary tract infection. *Clin Ther* 1982;4:5.
24. Kaslowski S, Radford N, Kincaid-Smith P. Crystalline and macrocrystalline nitrofurantoin in the treatment of urinary tract infection. *New Engl J Med* 1974;280:385.
25. Kursch ED, Mostyn EM, Persky L. Nitrofurantoin pulmonary complications. *J Urol* 1975;113:392.
26. Stamm W. Epidemiology and therapy of urinary tract infection in women. *Urinary tract infection and pelvic inflammatory disease - consensus conference proceedings.* City: Publisher, 1994:2–6.
27. Bates TR, Sequeira JA, Tembo AV. The effect of food on nitrofurantoin absorption. *Clin Pharmacol Ther* 1974;16:63.
28. Stamey TA, Nemay NJ, Higgens M. The clinical use of nalidixic acid: a review and some observations. *Invest Urol* 1969;6:582.
29. Swinney JL. Nalidixic acid. *Practitioner* 1964;192:1.
30. Slade DA. A clinical trial of nalidixic acid in thirty-three patients with urinary tract infections in general practive. *Brit J Urol* 1963;35:125.
31. Anonymous. Adverse effects of drugs commonly used in the treatment of urinary tract infections: a report from the Australian Drug Evaluation Committee. *Med J Aust* 1972; 1:435.
32. Gibson GR. A clinical appraisal of methenamine hippurate in urinary tract infection. *Med J Aust* 1970;1:167.
33. Greenfield W, Berg R, Moore R. Determination of urine formaldehyde following administration of methenamine salts. *Clin Chem* 1969;15:3.
34. Selwyn S. The evolution of the broad-spectrum penicillins. *J Antimicrob Chemother* 1982;9(Suppl B):23.
35. Eliopoulos GM. The penicillins. In: Peterson PK, Verhoef J, eds.*The antimicrobial agents annual 3.* Amsterdam: Elsevier Science Publishers BV; 1988:1–35.
36. Wright A, Wilkowske C. The penicillins. *Mayo Clin Proc* 1991;66:1047.
37. Amoxicillin. *Med Lett Drugs Ther* 1974;19:49.
38. Bang N, Kammer R. Hematologic complications associated with beta-lactam antibiotics. *Rev Infect Dis* 1983;5(Suppl 2):S380.
39. Dossetor J. Drug interactions with oral contraceptives. *Brit Med J* 1975;4:467.
40. Gould IM, Wise R. Beta-lactamase inhibitors. In: Peterson PK, Verhoef J, eds.*The antimicrobial agents annual 3.* Amsterdam: Elsevier Science Publishers BV; 1988:63–76.
41. Gustaferro C, Steckelberg J. Cephalosporin antimicrobial agents and related compounds. *Mayo Clin Proc* 1991;66:1064.
42. Neu HC. The new beta-lactamase stable cephalosporins. *Ann Intern Med* 1982;97:408.
43. Portier H, Chalopin SM, Freysz M, et al. Interaction between cephalosporins and alcohol. *Lancet* 1980;2:263.
44. Prentice RD, Wu LR, Gehlbach SH, Hanlon JT, Clapp-Channing NE. Treatment of lower urinary tract infections with single dose trimethoprim-sulfamethoxazole. *J Fam Pract* 1985;20:551.
45. Seidmon EJ, et al. Treatment of recurrent urinary tract infection with norfloxacin versus trimethoprim-sulfamethoxazole. *Urology* 1990;35:187.
46. Schaeffer AJ, Flynn S. Jones J. Comparison of cinoxacin and trimethoprim-sulfamethoxazole in the treatment of urinary tract infections. *J Urol* 1981;125:825.
47. Tolkoff-Rubin NE, et al. Single dose therapy with trimethoprim-sulfamethoxazole for urinary tract infection in women. *Rev Infect Dis* 1982;4:444.
48. Finn SD, et al. Trimethoprim-sulfamethoxazole for acute dysuria in women: a single-dose or 10-day course: a double-blind, randomized trial. *Ann Intern Med* 1988;108:350.
49. Cockerill F. Trimethoprim-sulfamethoxazole. *Mayo Clin Proc* 1991;66:1260.
50. Patel RB, Welling PG. Clinical pharmacokinetics of trimethoprim-sulfamethoxazole. *Clin Pharmacokinet* 1980;5:405.
51. Jick H. Adverse reactions to trimethoprim-sulfamethoxazole in hospitalized patients. *Rev Infect Dis* 1982;4:426.
52. Frish JM. Clinical experience with adverse reactions to trimethoprim-sulfamethoxazole. *J Infect Dis* 1973;128(Suppl):607.
53. Lawson DH, Paice BJ. Adverse reactions to trimethoprim-sulfamethoxazole. *Rev Infect Dis* 1982;4:429.

54. Gossius G, Vorland L. A randomized comparison of high-dose versus three-day and ten-day therapy with trimethoprim-sulfamethoxazole for acute cystitis in women. *Scand J Infect Dis* 1984;16:374.
55. Brumfitt W, Smith GW, Hamilton-Miller JMT, Gargan RA. A clinical comparison between Macrodantin and trimethoprim for prophylaxis in women with recurrent urinary tract infections. *J Antimicrob Agents and Chemother* 1985;16:111.
56. Labbe J. Comparison of two methods of trimethoprim-sulfamethoxazole prophylaxis of urinary tract infection in children. *Can Med Assoc J* 1984;131:1229.
57. Jaffe HS, Abrams DI, Ammann AJ, Lewis BJ, Golden JA. Complications of co-trimoxazole in treatment of AIDS-associated Pneumocystis carinii pneumonia in homosexual men. *Lancet* 1983;2:1109.
58. Wofsy CB. Use of trimethoprim-sulfamethoxazole in the treatment of Pneumocystis carinii pneumonitis in patients with acquired immunodeficiency syndrome. *Rev Infect Dis* 1987;9(Suppl 2):S184.
59. Appel GB, Neu HC. The nephrotoxicity of antimicrobial agents. *New Engl J Med* 1974;14:784.
60. Williams DN. Tetracyclines. In: Peterson PK, Verhoef J, eds. *The antimicrobial agents annual 3.* Amsterdam: Elsevier Science Publishers BV; 1988:218.
61. Neu HC. A symposium on the tetracyclines: a major appraisal. *Bull N Y Acad Med* 1978;54:141.
62. Smilack JD, Wilson WR, Cockerill FR. Tetracyclines, chloramphenicol, erythromycin, clindamycin and metronidazole. *Mayo Clin Proc* 1991;66:1270.
63. Kuzucu EY. Methoxyflurane, tetracycline and renal failure. *JAMA* 1970;211:1162.
64. Chopra I, Howe TGB. Bacterial resistance to the tetracyclines. *Microbiol Rev* 1978;42:707.
65. Williams JD. Aztreonam. In: Peterson PK, Verhoef J, eds. *The antimicrobial agents annual 3.* Amsterdam: Elsevier Science Publishers BV; 1988:51.
66. Childs SJ. Aztreonam in the treatment of urinary tract infection. *Am J Med* 1985;78(Suppl 2A):44.
67. Swabb EA, Jenkins SA, Muir JG. Summary of worldwide clinical trials of aztreonam in patients with urinary tract infections. *Rev Infect Dis* 1985;7(Suppl 4):S772.
68. Madsen PO, Nielsen KT, Graversen PH. Aztreonam: critical evaluation of the first monobactam antibiotic in treatment of urinary tract infections. *J Urol* 1988;140:925.
69. Newman TJ, Dreslinski GR, Tadros SS. Safety profile of aztreonam in clinical trials. *Rev Infect Dis* 1985;7(Suppl 4):S650.
70. Cypress BK. Patient's reasons for visiting physicians: national ambulatory medical care survey, United States, 1977–1978. Hyattsville, Maryland: National Center for Health Statistics; 1981; DHSS publication No. (PHS)82-1717. (*Vital and health statistics*; series 13; No. 56.)

Antibiotic Therapy in Urology,
edited by S. Grant Mulholland, M.D.,
Lippincott-Raven Publishers, Philadelphia © 1996.

Chapter 10

Errors in Antimicrobial Use and Reasons for Treatment Failure

David T. Uehling and John V. Kryger

Division of Urology, University of Wisconsin Hospitals and Clinics, Madison, Wisconsin 53792-3236

Previous chapters in this book have dealt with many of the important issues concerning the use of antibiotics for urinary tract infection (UTI). Described in these chapters are many of the caveats about inappropriate or unsuccessful use of antibiotics. In order to discuss errors in antimicrobial use further, we have chosen to present illustrative cases taken from our own practice. These cases describe patients for whom we feel the best treatment was not used by us or our colleagues. Obviously, all errors cannot be prevented and antibiotic use will not always be successful, even when the best principles and practice are applied. Errors in duration of therapy, route of administration, and antibiotic selection are presented. Other errors resulted from clinical situations in which infections were not present at the time but in which UTI might have been anticipated to occur and warrant prophylaxis. These involved prophylaxis for neurogenic bladder disease, prostate biopsy, transurethral resection of the prostate, and prophylaxis during pregnancy. Prevention of infection-related calculi in patients with urinary diversion remains difficult. Some errors in antimicrobial use emanated from expecting antibiotics to do too much, as in cases in which prophylaxis was not effective in the presence of an anatomic abnormality and surgery was required before prophylaxis could be effective. Errors of omission can occur as well as errors of commission. Illustrative of this is our case in which a child developed a renal abscess because the diagnosis of a genitourinary infection was not made until later in the clinical course. Since we all learn by our own experience and that of others, we hope these illustrative cases will bring up some of the situations in which errors in antimicrobial use can be lessened in the future. Finally, every effort needs to be made not to give antibiotics to every patient at risk and to give them only for the minimal duration needed to be effective. This chapter and others in this book and the UTI literature repeatedly return to the serious problem of antibiotic overuse, leading to selection of antibiotic-resistant urinary pathogens (1).

CASE 1

Short Duration of Treatment

A 3-year-old girl presented with a first episode of frequency, dysuria, and irritability. Physical examination was negative. A clean voided urine was obtained and showed pyuria. Methylene blue-stained smear of the urinary sediment showed short rods suggestive of *Escherichia coli* (2). The patient was placed on trimethoprim/sulfamethoxazole (TMP/SMX) 1 tsp twice daily. Since the child seemed to improve rapidly, the mother stopped the medicine after 2 days of a recommended 10-day course. The child returned 1 week later for ultrasonographic imaging of kidneys and bladder; results were normal. However, the child again was irritable and had continuing urinary frequency. Urinalysis with stained smear of the sediment again showed short rods suggestive of *E. coli*. The urine culture and sensitivity again showed pansensitive *E. coli*. The mother was instructed to administer a full 10-day course, and the child was well when seen 1 week after stopping the TMP/SMX.

This case illustrates the concept that short-course antibiotic therapy for urinary tract infections in children may not be as effective as a longer course. This was seen in a child who had the appropriate imaging evaluation for a first infection, which revealed no abnormality (3). Antibiotic therapy in such an uncomplicated case should be given for 7 to 10 days, even though not all series have seen a clear difference (4,5). Ruberto et al. (6) found no difference in 3- vs. 10-day treatment courses in 110 children age 5 to 12 years of age. Relapses occurred in 13.8% of the patients given treatment for 3 days and 15.4% given treatment for 10 days. Madrigal and colleagues (7) randomly assigned 132 children with acute urinary tract infection to receive TMP/SMX in one dose only, two doses daily for 3 days, or three doses daily for 7 days. The patient characteristics, etiologic agents, and frequency of radiographic abnormalities were similar for the treatment groups. The differences in rate of recurrent urinary tract infection between the single-dose (20.5%) regimen compared with the 3-day (5.6%) and 7-day (8%) regimens were statistically significant. These authors concluded that a single dose of TMP/SMX was inadequate treatment for infants and children with acute urinary tract infection. Moffatt et al. (8) reviewed 14 published clinical trials of short-course (4 days or less) vs. conventional (7- to 10-day) antibiotic therapy for urinary tract infection in children. Two studies found short-course antibiotic therapy significantly less effective than conventional therapy, and the remaining 12 had insufficient sample size to warrant the conclusion that the two therapies were equivalent. These authors concluded that there was not good evidence to warrant the use of short-course antibiotic therapy in children. It is our practice not to use single-dose or 3-day therapy for acute UTIs in infants and children.

CASE 2

Inappropriate Route

A 7-month-old girl presented to her family doctor with fever, lassitude, and vomiting. There were no physical findings, but a urinary tract infection was suspected. Urinalysis showed pyuria and bacteriuria, and TMP/SMX suspension twice daily was started empirically. Two days after initiation of therapy, urine culture and sensitivity showed *E. coli* sensitive to TMP/SMX. However, the child continued to vomit and have a fever to 39°C. Renal and bladder ultrasonography performed on admission to the hospital showed right hydroureteronephrosis and a filling defect in the bladder compatible with a ureterocele (Figs. 1,2). After 5 days of in-

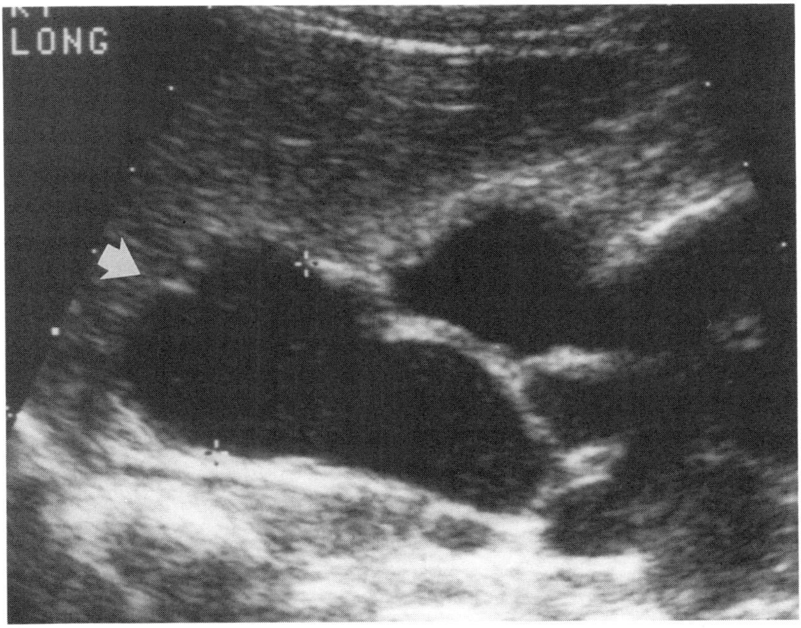

FIG. 1. Case 2: Longitudinal ultrasonographic view of right upper pole hydronephrosis (*arrow*).

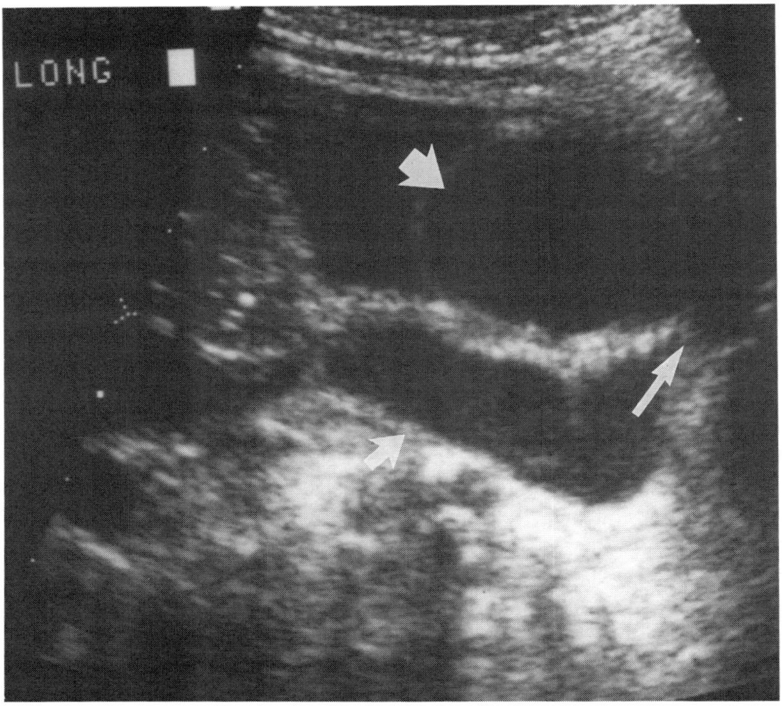

FIG. 2. Case 2: Longitudinal ultrasonographic view of dilated upper pole ureter (*small arrow*) entering ureterocele in bladder (*large arrow*).

travenous ampicillin and gentamicin, the patient underwent cystoscopy and needle retrograde pyelogram of the ureterocele, which showed a massively dilated ureter subserving the hydronephrotic upper pole. Another orifice was seen subserving the lower pole, and there was a single orifice on the left. The child underwent right heminephrectomy and made a good postoperative recovery, although she eventually required ureterocele repair with excision of the upper pole ureter and reimplantation of the lower pole ureter.

This case illustrates ineffective antibiotic use resulting from an inappropriate route of administration. While some children with febrile UTIs respond to oral antibiotics, children who are vomiting require parenteral antibiotic therapy. All toxic-appearing infants and children and all febrile infants without an apparent source should be considered for hospitalization and parenteral antibiotic therapy. Febrile infants 28 to 90 days defined as low-risk by clinical and laboratory criteria may be managed in selected cases as outpatients if close follow-up is assured (9). Older children with a fever of less than 39°C and a white blood cell count of less than 15,000/mm^3 may not need hospitalization. In febrile infants, it is important to rule out bacteremia and meningitis. The severity of the fever, the physical findings, the laboratory evaluation, and the social situation, including availability of medical care, taken together should constitute the criteria for admission for febrile UTIs. While an ultrasonogram was done relatively early in this child's clinical course, it could have been done even earlier and used to direct parenteral therapy. This is shown by a series in which the incidence of urinary tract infection in infants with a prenatal ultrasonographic diagnosis of hydronephrosis was assessed (10). After 13 boys with posterior urethral valves were excluded, 13 (3.1%) of 413 children presented with urinary tract infection within the first 6 months of life. Ten of the 13 were boys and 7 were not circumcised. The cause of hydronephrosis was reflux in 6, ureteropelvic junction obstruction in 6, and primary megaureter in 1. Amoxicillin-resistant bacteria were the causative organisms in 10 infants. Four categories of management failure were identified: (a) prenatal findings not communicated, (b) antibiotics not prescribed, (c) antibiotics prescribed but not administered, and (d) infection despite continuous antibiotic prophylaxis. Uncircumcised infants with reflux seemed to be at special risk for infection.

While gentamicin and ampicillin remain the gold standard in intravenous therapy of serious genitourinary infections, other intravenous and intramuscular antibiotics have also been used with good success (1). Ceftriaxone can be given as a once- or twice-daily intramuscular treatment of serious bacterial infections in children. Frenkel (11) reported that the infections of all 14 children treated empirically with ceftriaxone for a urinary tract source were clinically and bacteriologically resolved. Ceftriaxone therapy has less effectiveness (78% bacteriologic cure rate) when used for gram-positive infections. A once-daily intramuscular dose may be useful for outpatient management. Most families can bring their child to their physician's office or the emergency room for the daily intramuscular injection, which obviates the need for intravenous access. In another series, outpatient or inpatient treatment with empiric intramuscular administration of ceftriaxone (50 mg/kg/day) was generally effective when carried out after cultures of blood, urine, and cerebrospinal fluid were monitored (12). The children treated as outpatients needed to have a caretaker available by telephone and had to return for daily outpatient visits. Other candidates for outpatient treatment were those children who did not appear ill, who had no source of fever detected on physical examination, who had a peripheral leukocyte count of less than 20×10^9 cells/L, who had a cerebrospinal fluid leukocyte count of less than 10^6/L, and who did not have measurable urinary leukocyte esterase. Some children with serious sepsis later required a different course of antimicrobial therapy, and children with meningitis received twice-daily intravenous regimens. Parenteral therapy with ceftriaxone does not require peak or trough serum levels, although some monitoring of renal function should be carried out (13). When ceftriaxone is given intramuscularly, buffered lidocaine is the preferable diluent (14). For hospitalized patients who need parenteral therapy and are allergic to penicillins and cephalosporins, aztreonam may be a suitable antibiotic (15). Aztreonam provides high urine levels and is highly active against most gram-negative bacteria and some *Pseudomonas* strains. Patients can be switched to an orally administered antimicrobial agent once they have stopped vomiting. For the seriously ill and vomiting patient, varying parenteral antibiotic regimens need to be considered.

CASE 3

Inappropriate Choice for Clinical Situation

A 20-year-old college student presented with frequency and dysuria that had started the evening before her clinic visit. She reported being sexually active, taking birth control pills for contraception, and having had several previous UTI episodes for which antibiotics of unknown type were prescribed. Physical examination showed no flank or suprapubic tenderness. Urinalysis showed between 15 and 20 WBCs per high-power field, and methylene blue-stained smear of the urinary sediment showed cocci in chains. The patient had previously been treated with TMP/SMX and asked for that again. However, urine culture grew out *Enterococcus faecalis* resistant to sulfonamides. The patient returned unimproved 24 hours later and was switched to nitrofurantoin.

This case illustrates the increasing prevalence of UTIs caused by enterococci and *Staphylococcus* species. Both tend to occur in sexually active young women and in patients who have had a previous course of antibiotics or urologic instrumentation (16). In recent years, the pathogenic potential of enterococci and *Staphylococcus* species for the urinary tract has been convincingly shown. Isolation of species of enterococci from patients with urinary tract infections rose from 4% in 1971 to 12.6% in 1989 in hospital patients and from 2–5.6% in general-practice patients (17). Enterococci are indistinguishable from streptococci on Gram stain—hence their original classification as part of the group D streptococci under the Lancefield scheme. DNA restriction patterns have clearly demonstrated that they should be classified separately (18). The most important species in the genus is *E. faecalis*, but *E. faecium* has become a major hospital problem because of its vancomycin and ampicillin resistance (17). While enterococci may translocate from the gastrointestinal tract to mesenteric nodes, most clinical studies suggest that enterococci are spread from patient to patient in the hospital (19). The usefulness of the methylene blue-stained smear of the urinary sediment becomes apparent when dealing with coccal urinary bacteria (2). While a Gram stain shows the difference between gram-positive and gram-negative cocci, the methylene blue-stained smear shows the cocci, which are probably enterococci if in chains and staphylococci if in clumps. Urinary tract infections caused by enterococci can be treated with penicillin or ampicillin alone as long as the infecting strains are not lactamase-producing. The majority of outpatient enterococcal UTI isolates remain susceptible to nitrofurantoin, which is the preferable agent for UTIs if these organisms are suspected (19). At the current time in our hospital, the antibiotic sensitivity for all enterococcal species is ampicillin 81%, vancomycin 99%, nitrofurantoin 100%, and quinolones 42%. UTIs caused by *S. saprophyticus* also are becoming more frequent and often involve the kidney. In one series of 57 women with staphylococcal urinary tract infections, the clinical symptoms suggested renal involvement in 29 patients (20). Renal concentrating ability was also reduced during the course of these infections. Patients with renal calculi had a high incidence of persistent growth of *S. saprophyticus* despite treatment with antibiotics to which the organisms were sensitive *in vitro*. This case illustrates one method (stained smear of urinary sediment) that can facilitate antibiotic selection at the time of the patient's clinic visit.

CASE 4

Development of Antibiotic Resistance

A 65-year-old woman with long-standing diabetes mellitus presented with recurrent UTI. Evaluation included a normal kidney and bladder ultrasonogram, normal cystoscopy, and an elevated residual urine. On her first urologic visit, the urinalysis showed heavy pyuria and bacteriuria with short rods suggestive of *E. coli*. A quinolone was prescribed, but the *E. coli* was shown 48 hours later to be resistant to the quinolones in our hospital panel. The patient was switched to nitrofurantoin, to which the *E. coli* remained sensitive. The infection cleared and she was placed on low-dose nitrofurantoin as prophylaxis.

The ineffectiveness of the first antibiotic selected in this case illustrates the acquisition of urinary tract infections caused by quinolone-resistant *E. coli*. For UTI, the different quinolones are thought to be equally effective and interchangeable. While this patient did not know which antibiotics she had previously received, it is likely that she had been previously treated with a quinolone. She also had the predisposing anatomic abnormality of elevated residual urine characteristic of a diabetic. While it was not definitely an error to prescribe a quinolone as first-line treatment in this patient, the overuse of quinolone antibiotics is one factor in the growing resistance of gram-negative bacteria to the quinolone group of antibiotics. In a review of risk factors for acquisition of quinolone-resistant *E. coli* infections, patients with quinolone-resistant *E. coli* had a greater prevalence of asymptomatic bacteriuria and had more of a history of relapse after previous regimens (21). Our preference for first-line treatment of uncomplicated outpatient UTI would be TMP/SMX or nitrofurantoin. In our hospital at the current time, *E. coli* sensitivity is 67% for ampicillin, 93% for cefazolin, 96% for gentamicin, 87% for TMP/SMX, 99% for nitrofurantoin, 95% for the quinolones, and 80% for tetracycline. At one time it was uncommon to encounter quinolone-resistant *E. coli*, but this is no longer the case. While we did not do *E. coli* serotyping or assessment of bacterial virulence factors, studies of others have shown that certain *E. coli* serotypes and "adhesins" are associated with increased pathogenicity (22). *E. coli* restriction fragment length polymorphism patterns, plasmid profiles, and antimicrobial susceptibility patterns generally remain similar for patients who fail treatment and show different patterns for those who become reinfected (23). While these assays are not available for average clinical practice, they reveal why bacteria become antibiotic-resistant and may indicate ways to avoid or slow the development of antibiotic resistance. Antibiotic selection can best be made with accurate assessment of the clinical situation and updated information on current antibiotic sensitivities.

CASE 5

Prophylaxis in Pregnancy

A 26-year-old woman was referred in the 24th week of her second pregnancy for three UTIs occurring over the past 6 weeks. Urinalysis again showed pyuria and bacteriuria. Urine culture and sensitivity revealed *E. coli* sensitive to TMP/SMX and nitrofurantoin but resistant to cephalosporins. Renal ultrasonography showed minimal upper-tract dilatation. The patient was treated with nitrofurantoin macrocrystals 100 mg qid for 3 days and then put on a regimen of 50 mg of nitrofurantoin to be taken postcoitally. The remainder of the pregnancy was without any further UTIs, and she delivered a healthy term baby.

UTIs during pregnancy continue to present a difficult management problem. Asymptomatic or symptomatic UTIs during pregnancy can result in temporary or permanent renal damage in the pregnant woman (24). UTI can also have serious deleterious effects on the fetus, including retardation of intrauterine growth, prematurity, and increased risk of perinatal death. *E. coli* remains the predominant urinary pathogen in these infections, but *Gardnerella vaginalis* can be the urinary pathogen more commonly than would be expected. Staphylococci, enterococci, and *Pro-*

teus and *Pseudomonas* species increase in patients who have received prior antibiotic treatment. Choosing the best antibiotic for UTI treatment or prophylaxis during pregnancy requires both maternal and fetal consideration. Penicillin and cephalosporins are probably the safest and most-used antibiotics in the pregnant patient (25). Tetracycline and erythromycin are associated with an increase of hepatotoxicity in pregnant women and should be avoided. While TMP/SMX may be associated with an increased risk of maternal megaloblastic anemia because of its antifolate action in combination with increased nutritional requirements of the pregnancy, this agent has also been widely used. For fetal considerations, chloramphenicol and tetracycline are contraindicated. Sulfonamides cannot be handled by the neonatal liver, so their preterm administration can lead to kernicterus in the baby. Nitrofurantoin is safe for use in pregnant women and is thought not to cause increased risk of teratogenic or other adverse fetal effects. There is not sufficient information to justify the use of short-course therapy in pregnancy, and a 7-day course should be recommended (26). Acute pyelonephritis complicates 1% of pregnancies, so renal ultrasonography should be carried out after a first UTI and possibly repeated to rule out progressive upper-tract dilatation and calculi.

Since UTI prevention is particularly important during pregnancy, low-dose prophylaxis has been tried with several regimens. One study evaluated 200 patients following hospital admission for an acute episode of pyelonephritis during pregnancy (27). Recurrent pyelonephritis occurred in 7% of patients receiving prophylaxis vs. 8% of those receiving only close surveillance. This study questioned the need for prophylaxis and emphasized the beneficial effects of close surveillance with urine cultures. In this high-risk population; patients with gram-negative bacilluria of less than 10^5 colonies per milliliter were at greater risk of developing symptomatic recurrences. Another study showed that screening and active treatment of asymptomatic bacteriuria caused reduction in the incidence of pyelonephritis from 1.8–0.6% (28). Postcoital prophylaxis consisting of a single dose either of 250 mg of cephalexin or 50 mg of nitrofurantoin macrocrystals has been used effectively; 30 UTIs occurred in 39 pregnant women before the use of a postcoital regimen, and only 1 occurred after this regimen (29). UTIs in pregnancy require careful monitoring and may be managed by judicious prophylaxis.

CASE 6

Prophylaxis Failure Caused by Anatomic Abnormality

An 8-year-old boy underwent evaluation for recurrent febrile UTIs. The imaging findings included an absent right kidney, marked caliectasis and dilatation of the left collecting system, and high-grade left vesicoureteral reflux (Figs. 3,4). Cystoscopy showed no other abnormality except for an absent right ureteral orifice and a laterally placed scalloped left ureteral orifice. The child was kept on single or double UTI prophylaxis with TMP/SMX and nitrofurantoin suspension but required two hospitalizations during each of 2 years because of febrile episodes of left pyelonephritis. The organisms grown on these four occasions included resistant *E. coli* twice, *Klebsiella* once, and enterococci once. Because of these episodes of breakthrough pyelonephritis, the child underwent left ureteroneocystostomy with ureteral tapering and psoas hitch. Postoperative evaluation showed resolution of the left vesicoureteral reflux and better bladder emptying. The patient is being kept on TMP/SMX prophylaxis while his clinical course is followed.

Prophylactic antibiotics may be ineffective in the presence of one or more UTI susceptibility factors. Vesicoureteral reflux is one factor predisposing children to ascending recurrent urinary tract infections (30).

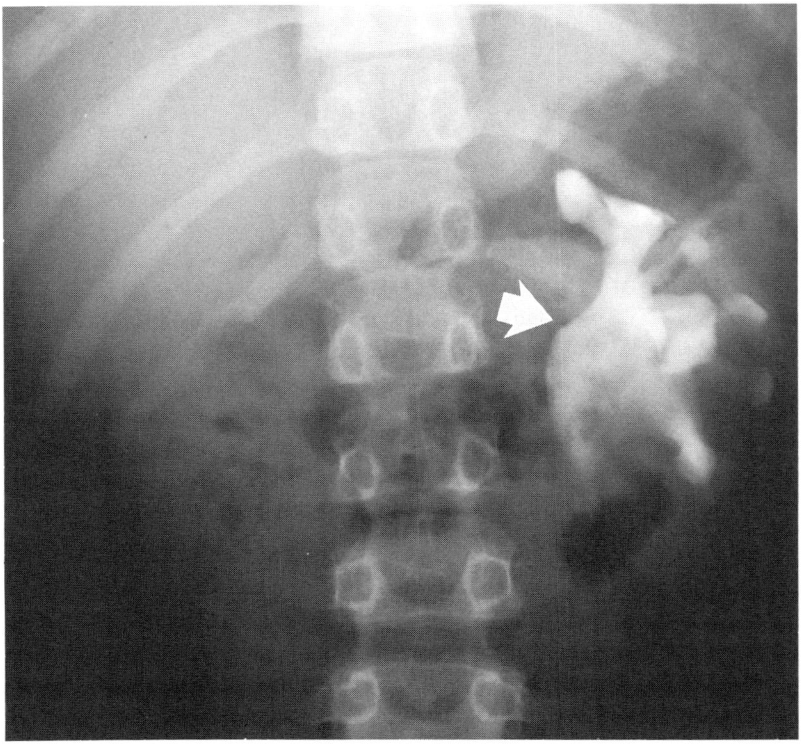

FIG. 3. Case 6: Intravenous pyelogram showing dilated left collecting system (*arrow*) and absent kidney on right.

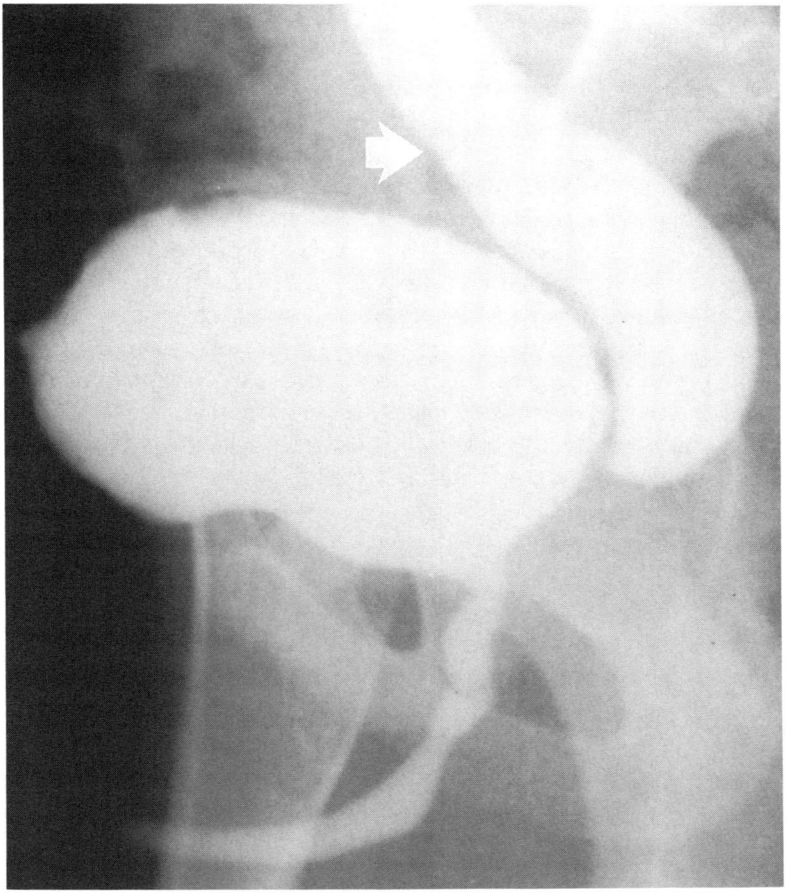

FIG. 4. Case 6: Voiding cystourethrogram showing high-grade reflux into left ureter (*arrow*) and radiographically normal urethra.

Other factors that may lead to ascending infections are changes in introital flora, nonlaminar flow in the urethra, deficiency in the bladder mucin layer, differences in receptors on bladder epithelial cells, low urinary antibody, bladder abnormalities such as diverticula, uncoordinated emptying of the bladder, ascent of bacteria into the ureter without radiographic reflux, and the known heightened susceptibility of the kidney to bacterial infection. Single or double prophylaxis may prevent many ascending infections even when reflux is present (31). In one study of 94 children with febrile UTIs evaluated by dimercaptosuccinic acid (DMSA) renal scans, 62 children (66%) had photon-deficient areas consistent with acute pyelonephritis (32). Vesicoureteral reflux was demonstrated in 29 (31% of the total group) and in 23 (37%) of the 62 patients with DMSA evidence of pyelonephritis. While reflux is not the only susceptibility factor to be considered in groups of children with acute pyelonephritis, it is an important one that may require surgery. It is difficult to know which children with high-grade reflux will have breakthrough infections and which infections may lead to significant pyelonephritis and renal scarring. In the case report described above, there seemed to be clear evidence of breakthrough febrile infections even though the mother was very conscientious in giving her child daily single or double prophylaxis (31). The incidence of renal failure attributable to vesicoureteral reflux is also not well defined. In one family we studied, four of six siblings manifested vesicoureteral reflux, but reflux could not be demonstrated in preceding or succeeding generations of the family (33). Within this family, one of six siblings developed renal failure and later required renal transplantation. An anatomic abnormality such as vesicoureteral reflux may require surgical correction before antibiotic prophylaxis can be effective.

CASE 7

Prophylaxis for Open Surgery

A 65-year-old woman was a kidney donor to her daughter with end-stage renal failure caused by diabetes mellitus. The donor's preliminary evaluation showed a normal intravenous pyelogram, single arteries bilaterally on renal arteriogram, and a creatinine clearance of 80 ml/min. Left donor nephrectomy was carried out without peritoneal or pleural entry, and systemic antibiotics were not given. Wound irrigation with bacitracin and gentamicin solution was carried out as the muscle and fascial layers were closed. The subcutaneous tissue was closed with a 4-0 polyglycolate subcuticular suture. An indwelling bladder catheter was used and removed on the morning of the first postoperative day. The urine culture thereafter remained negative. The wound seemed to be healing well and the patient was discharged on the fifth postoperative day. Two weeks after going home and 3 weeks after the operative date, the incision became red, tender, and swollen in its midsection. The area of maximum induration was opened and a small amount of yellowish pus was allowed to drain. A small Penrose drain was placed in the subcutaneous abscess, which was superficial to the muscle and fascial layers. *Staphylococcus aureus* grew from the wound culture. This organism was sensitive to amoxicillin, which was given orally for 5 days. The Penrose drain was removed and there was continued healing of the incision. Thereafter, the patient's convalescence was uneventful.

The use of systemic antibiotics for open urologic surgery remains controversial. In a recent article covering antimicrobial prophylaxis for surgical wounds of all types, a wound infection rate of 10% or less was given for clean-contaminated procedures in which there is transection of gastrointestinal, genitourinary, or biliary tracts (such as donor nephrectomy) (34). Use of antibiotics in clean-contaminated surgical procedures is appropriate in certain instances, such as insertion of a prosthesis, in which there is a low infection rate but high morbidity (35). Extension of antibiotic coverage to other categories of clean wounds should be limited to patients with two or more of established risk factors. Cefazolin remains the mainstay of prophylactic therapy. If surgical prophylaxis is used, it should be given 2 hours before the procedure (36). The duration of therapy possibly can be limited to the intraoperative period; this has been reported to be equally effective as 24- to 48-hour coverage (37). *E. coli*, *Klebsiella*, *Proteus*, and *Enterobacter* species are the primary urinary pathogens in urologic wound infections. The wound infection is from the same organism that is infecting the urinary tract, if such is the case. In our recent review of complications following living-related donor nephrectomy, 4% of 681 patients developed a wound infection (38). These patients did not receive systemic prophylactic antibiotics but did receive antibiotic wound irrigation during closure. The use of systemic antibiotics during clean or clean-contaminated open urologic procedures such as living-donor nephrectomy probably can be considered a judgment choice. We have continued not to not systemic antibiotics in our attempts to lower antibiotic use. While we would not consider this case an error in antibiotic use, others might, and it is presented to illustrate a situation in which a rationale can be made for both giving and not giving systemic prophylaxis for open urologic surgery.

CASE 8

Delay of Diagnosis

A 6-year-old boy presented with fever, chills, and left flank pain. Urine culture showed pyuria and bacteriuria. The urine culture grew out *E. faecalis*, and the child was placed on intravenous ampicillin and gentamicin. Renal ultrasonography showed a left intrarenal abscess, and this was confirmed by abdominal CT, which also showed a dilated left renal pelvis (Fig. 5). On intravenous antibiotics the abscess rapidly cleared, and no intervention was required. On further questioning, the patient described several unexplained febrile illnesses associated with abdominal pain over the preceding months. On one of these occasions he had had a urinalysis that was negative. On the other occasions a urinalysis had not been carried out. Following the diagnosis of the abscess, voiding cystourethrogram showed no vesicoureteral reflux or urethral abnor-

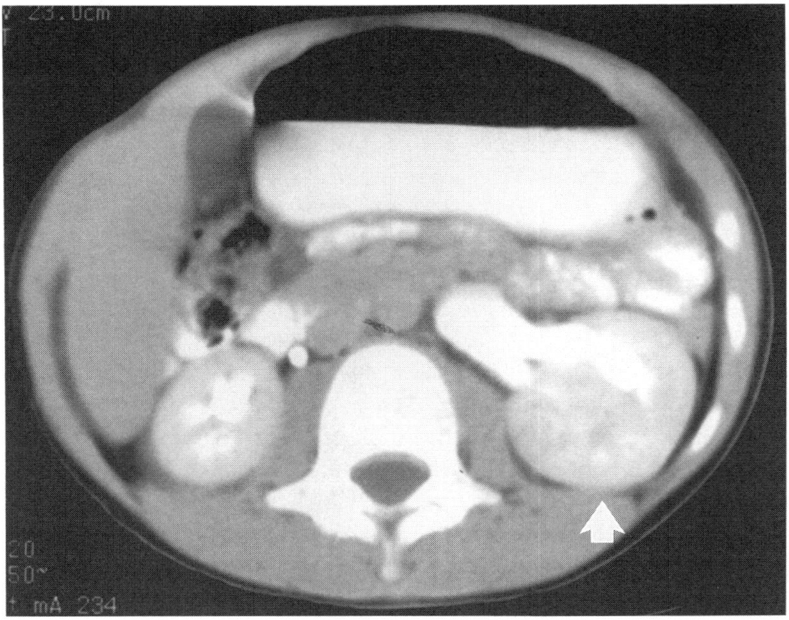

FIG. 5. Case 8: Abdominal CT showing left renal abscess (*large arrow*).

malities. Intravenous pyelogram showed a dilated left renal pelvis with a duplicating collection system (Fig. 6). Nucleotide scan showed 55% function on the right and 45% on the left. The $T^{1}/_{2}$ was 8 minutes for the right kidney and 9 minutes for the left kidney. While this child did not have classic ureteropelvic junction obstruction, the dilated collecting system on the left side probably indicates the reason for his development of a renal abscess.

In this case, the error in antibiotic use was an error of omission through a delay in making an early diagnosis. Without timely treatment, renal infection can lead to abscess formation. In a review of renal abscesses, Fowler and Perkins (39) reported a mean age of 51 years and intrarenal location in 26%. Predisposing causes such as diabetes mellitus, calculi, ureteral obstruction, and immunosuppression were usually present. The symptoms usually consisted of fever, abdominal pain, chills, and irritative voiding symptoms. *Escherichia coli*, *Proteus mirabilis*, *Klebsiella pneumoniae*, and other Enterobacteriaceae were the usual causative organisms. Bacteria in some patients were isolated only in blood cultures, which were positive in 41% of patients. Bacteria in other patients were isolated only from the urine, and some patients did not have any positive bacterial identification. An intravenous

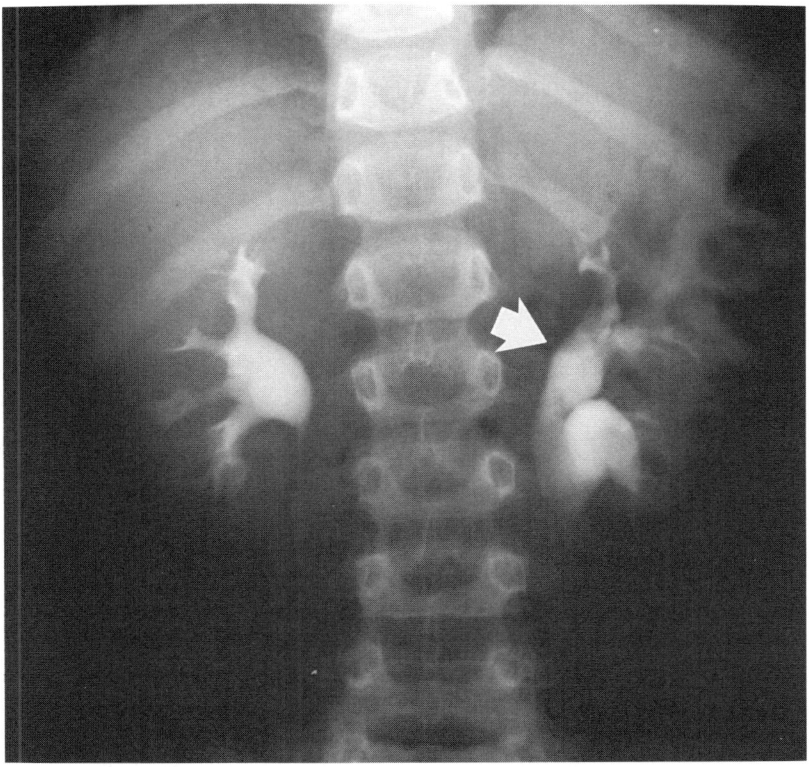

FIG. 6. Case 8: Intravenous pyelogram showing dilated left renal pelvis (*arrow*) and duplicated upper collecting system.

pyelogram or renal ultrasonogram usually revealed the mass lesion, and this was confirmed by CT later in the series. Ninety-three percent of these patients had an interventional procedure to drain the abscess, but in recent years fewer patients have required intervention. Four patients treated in the series died following delay in diagnosis. In a pediatric series, the role of anaerobic bacteria was emphasized in perinephric and renal abscesses (40). In 10 children, 20 organisms were recovered; 8 were aerobic or facultative bacteria, and 12 were anaerobic bacteria. Aerobic or facultative bacteria only were recovered in one patient, anaerobic only in 2, and mixed aerobic and anaerobic bacteria in 7. More common than a renal abscess is renal scarring attributable to a delay in diagnosis. In 50 of 52 children followed in a randomized prospective controlled trial of medical vs. surgical management of reflux, a delay in diagnosis was primarily held responsible for the degree of renal scarring seen (41). Increased awareness and earlier diagnosis remain a mainstay in effective antibiotic use for UTI.

CASE 9

Management of Asymptomatic Bacteriuria

A 35-year-old white man had incurred a C5-6 spinal cord injury at age 18 and now presented with asymptomatic bacteriuria. He had not been able to carry out intermittent catheterization and was now managing his bladder by voiding with suprapubic pressure into condom drainage. An intravenous pyelogram and renal ultrasonogram were normal and cystogram showed no reflux. His serum creatinine was stable at 1.1 mg/day and his residual urine was low. His asymptomatic bacteriuria had been caused by many different organisms, and attempts to sterilize the urine in the past had been unsuccessful. On two occasions during the past year urine cultures had shown *Pseudomonas aeruginosa* resistant to most antibiotics. Intravenous gentamicin had been given during an inpatient hospitalization in the rehabilitative care unit, but asymptomatic bacteriuria promptly recurred. Most recently the patient has remained asymptomatic, has been kept off antibiotics, and remains colonized with *Providencia* and *Pseudomonas* species.

This case illustrates the ineffectiveness of antibiotics in some situations and offers rationale for nontreatment in selected cases of asymptomatic bacteriuria. In adults, and in the absence of obstruction, vesicoureteral reflux, pregnancy, or impending urologic surgery, a rationale can be offered for selective nontreatment. Asymptomatic bacteriuria has not been associated with hypertension or deterioration of renal function in this clinical setting (19). There is no way to predict which patients will develop symptoms and no data to estimate how many will develop subsequent bacteremia (42). Antibiotic treatment in elderly women has been shown to result in reinfections with more highly resistant organisms (43). The purported increase in mortality in elderly bacteriuric patients more likely is caused by other associated fatal diseases such as cancer in men and the need for an indwelling catheter in women (44).

Patients on intermittent catheterization represent a similar situation. One prospective randomized study reported that patients with spinal cord injuries taking oral nitrofurantoin prophylaxis in combination with intravesical neomycin/polymyxin had fewer episodes of bacteriuria (45). However, another study found that patients on TMP/SMX prophylaxis had no difference in symptomatic urinary tract infections as compared with a placebo group (46). Symptomatic urinary tract infections occurred at the same rate whether asymptomatic infections were treated or not. Other series have reported that patients on intermittent catheterization using prophylactic antibiotics had fewer episodes of asymptomatic bacteria, but no fewer episodes of clinical urinary tract infections than patients who were not on antibiotics (47,48). All patients with indwelling catheters develop bacteriuria. If antibiotics are not given, the colonizing organisms may remain somewhat more sensitive to antibiotics (49,50). When a patient's catheter becomes dislodged or obstructed, sepsis can quickly develop. If patients have had periodic urine cultures and sensitivities but have not been treated, such septic episodes can be more easily treated when and if they occur.

In short-term catheterized patients, the findings are similar. In a study of 196 women undergoing elective gynecologic surgery, patients treated with prophylactic cefazolin had a decreased incidence of bacteriuria at the time of hospital discharge compared with the placebo group, but there was no difference in the febrile morbidity (51). Because increased drug resistance and drug toxicity were noted in the treated group, antimicrobial prophylaxis was not recommended for patients with noncritical underlying disease undergoing short-term catheterization. While quinolones have been reported to decrease the incidence of bacteriuria and symptomatic urinary tract infection after short-term indwelling catheterization, the presence of an indwelling urinary catheter also is a risk factor for the development of quinoline-resistant UTI (21,52). Bacterial biofilms are a barrier to antimicrobial penetration onto urinary catheters and represent a major reason for treatment failures. Organisms such as *Proteus* and *Pseudomonas* species are associated with a high propensity for biofilm growth (53,54). When antibiotics are to be utilized for patients with urinary catheters, they should be selected for their ability to penetrate biofilms (55,56). TMP/SMX may be ineffective against adherent uropathogens in biofilms and is associated in some cases with the emergence of drug-resistant species of *Pseudomonas* and enterococci (55). In carefully selected cases, asymptomatic bacteriuria can be judiciously not treated.

CASE 10

Calculi Secondary to Urease-Producing Organisms

An 81-year-old white woman underwent pelvic exenteration with ileal conduit urinary diversion for squamous cell carcinoma of the proximal urethra. Her ileal conduit became colonized with multiple organisms, including species of *Klebsiella*, *Enterobacter*, *Providencia*, and enterococci. No antibiotic therapy was given. An intravenous pyelogram in 1987 and subsequent yearly kidney, ureter, and bladder examinations demonstrated no evidence of calculi. The patient's ileal conduit subsequently became colonized with *Proteus mirabilis*, and she presented with fever, chills, and bacteremia caused by *Klebsiella pneumoniae* and *P. mirabilis*. A renal ultrasonogram demonstrated a right hydronephrosis and a large calculus. After nephrostomy tube placement

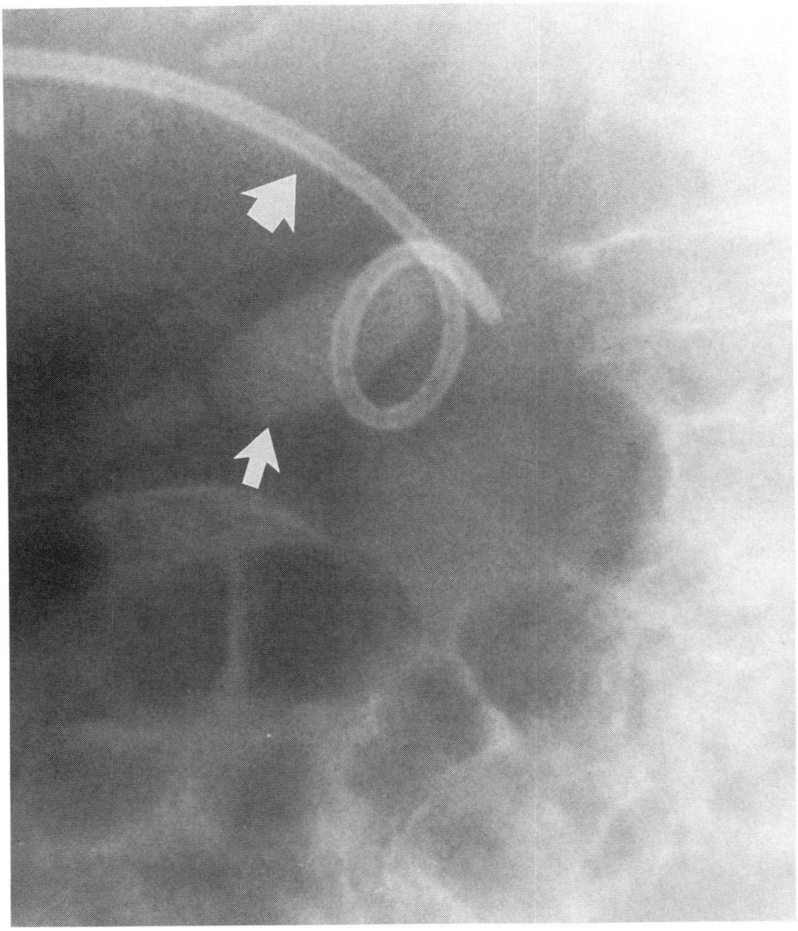

FIG. 7. Case 10: Percutaneous nephrostomy tube (*large arrow*) placed in right renal pelvis in proximity to large right renal calculi (*small arrow*).

and intravenous antibiotic therapy, she underwent percutaneous nephrolithotomy (Figs. 7,8). Analysis of the calculus fragments demonstrated a stone composition of 100% calcium phosphate. The nephrostomy tube was removed, and the patient's conduit continues to be colonized with nonurease-producing organisms.

UTIs caused by some urinary pathogens, especially *Proteus* and *Pseudomonas* species, may lead to development of urinary calculi. Failure to treat types of urinary tract colonization that more frequently lead to calculus formation can be considered an error in antimicrobial use. Reciprocally, the presence of infected stones is a reason for treatment failure in patients with chronic urinary tract infections. Infection-re-

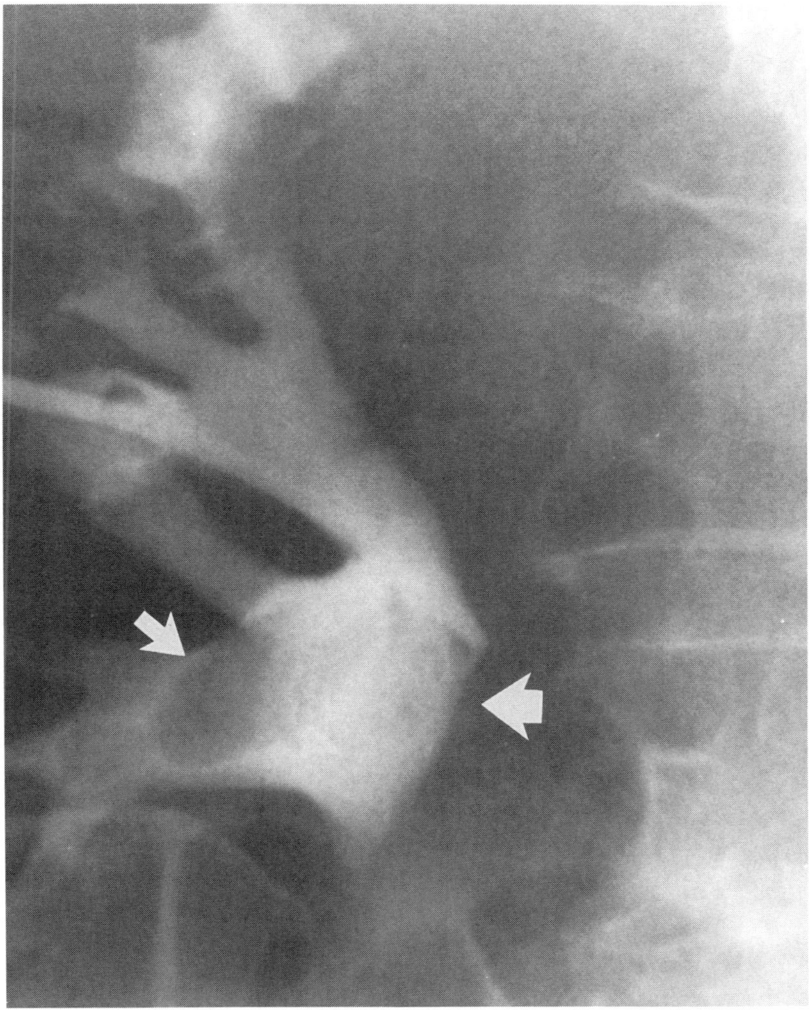

FIG. 8. Case 10: Right hydronephrosis (*large arrow*) caused by renal calculi seen as rounded filling defect (*small arrow*).

lated calculi in the urinary tract are almost always associated with infection by a urease-producing organism (57,58). Urease is produced by more than 45 different organisms, including *Proteus*, *Pseudomonas*, *Klebsiella*, *Providencia*, and *Staphylococcus* species. *Ureaplasma urealyticum* and *Corynebacterium urealyticum* are also urease producers that are difficult to culture in standard growth media. The presence of these organisms in a patient thought to be free of calculi is an indication for antibiotic therapy (59–61). Patients with spinal cord injuries, urinary diversion, and bladder augmentation have an increased incidence of urease-producing infections. Treatment of these infections requires careful use of sensitivity information from urine and the stone itself (62). The presence of infection-related stones ideally requires the removal of all of the stone material to clear the urinary tract infection. However, the use of antibiotics after extracorporeal shock wave lithotripsy (ESWL) may allow resolution of infection in patients with residual fragments of struvite stones (63,64). Inhibition of urease activity by quinolones, in addition to their antibacterial activity, may prevent the progression of urinary tract tissue damage and stone formation (65). The main goal of UTI treatment in the presence of calculi is removal of all calculi if possible and treatment of urease-producing bacteria when encountered. Treatment of urease-producing bacterial colonization, even in an otherwise asymptomatic patient, requires careful consideration.

CASE 11

Prophylaxis for Prostate Biopsy and Surgery

A 55-year-old man was referred for transrectal prostate biopsy because of an elevated prostate-specific antigen (PSA). The patient received prophylaxis with ciprofloxacin 500 mg orally twice daily for 3 days starting the evening prior to the biopsy. Prophylaxis was complicated by a rash and itching, but the patient had no postbiopsy UTI and the biopsy specimen was negative for cancer. Six months later the patient's PSA continued to rise and he underwent a repeated transrectal prostate biopsy utilizing TMP/SMX prophylaxis of one single-strength tablet twice a day for 3 days starting the evening prior to the biopsy. Two days after the biopsy, the patient presented to the emergency room with acute sepsis manifested by a fever to 39°C, shaking chills, nausea, and vomiting. The patient was admitted to the hospital for antibiotic therapy with ampicillin, gentamicin, and metronidazole. Urine and blood cultures were positive for *E. coli* that was resistant to TMP/SMX. The patient's fever subsided after a 3-day course, at which time he was changed to oral antibiotics for an additional 10-day course. Subsequent urine cultures were negative, and his biopsy specimens have remained negative.

This case demonstrates the challenges of antibiotic use for prostate biopsy and surgery. Eradication of bacteria from the prostate is hampered by poor penetrability of some antibiotics into the prostate. Meares (66) showed that high prostate antibiotic levels of drugs were achieved with rosaramicin, erythromycin, oleandomycin, clindamycin, and TMP. Rosaramicin and TMP exhibited the best in vitro activity against the gram-negative organisms that usually cause bacterial prostatitis. Secretory dysfunction during prostatitis causes secretions to become more alkaline and influences the passage of antibiotics into prostatic fluid. Quinolones reach high and long-lasting concentrations in prostatic and seminal fluid as well as prostate tissue (67–69). Prophylactic antibiotics should be administered preoperatively to uninfected as well as infected patients who undergo transurethral resection of the prostate (TURP) to prevent bacteremia (70–72). Single-dose preoperative ceftriazone has been reported to prevent UTI following TURP better than either TMP/SMX or no antibiotic (73). Short-term oral enoxacin has been shown to prevent bacteriuria in patients with sterile preoperative urine undergoing prostatectomy (74). Oral lomefloxacin has been shown to be equally efficacious and safe compared with parenteral cefotaxime in TURP prophylaxis (75). Prophylactic antibiotics seem well established for endoscopic surgery, although the route and duration of treatment will continue to be redefined.

The principles of antibiotic prophylaxis for prostate surgery act as guidelines for prostate biopsy prophylaxis. Bacteremia can be demonstrated in 73–100% of patients undergoing transrectal prostate biopsies when no antibiotic prophylaxis is utilized (76). The causative organisms in this bacteremia are *Bacteroides*, enterococci, and *E. coli* strains (77). Studies evaluating TMP/SMX prophylaxis in transrectal prostate biopsies have reported an incidence of febrile episodes in up to 32% of untreated patients (78). Quinolones have become the preferred antibiotic for prostate biopsy because they are lipid-soluble, not highly protein-bound, and highly soluble in an alkaline environment. Patients treated with prophylactic quinolones are reported to have an incidence of febrile episodes in 1–9% of cases and urinary tract infection in 4% of cases (79–82). Prophylactic antibiotics are indicated before prostate biopsy, and careful consideration is needed to provide the optimal regimen for each individual patient.

SUMMARY

These cases illustrate situations we have observed in which antibiotic use might have been improved. Some so-called "errors" might be considered judgment differences since antibiotic use will not always be successful. Prophylaxis is indicated for selected clinical situations but not for all genitourinary surgery. Some clinical situations cannot be resolved with antibiotics alone. Overuse of antibiotics might be considered the most serious and physician-remedial problem. We hope that these case presentations and discussions will stimulate critical thinking and promote continuing investigative efforts.

REFERENCES

1. Sobel JD, Kaye D. Urinary tract infections. In: Mandell GL, Bennett JE, Doln R., eds. *Principles and practice of infections and diseases.* New York: Churchill Livingstone; 1995:662–689.
2. Wear JB Jr. Correlation of pyuria, stained urine smear, urine culture and the uroscreen test. *J Urol* 1966;96:808–811.
3. MacKenzie JR, Fowler K, Hollman AS, Tappin D, Murphy AV, Beattie TJ, Azmy AF. The value of ultrasound in the child with an acute urinary tract infection. *Br J Urol* 1994;74:240–244.
4. Sherbotie JR, Cornfeld D. Management of urinary tract infections in children. *Med Clin North Am* 1991;75:327–328.
5. McCracken Jr GH. Diagnosis and management of acute urinary tract infections in infants and children. *J Infect Dis* 1987;6:107–112.
6. Ruberto U, D'Eufemia P, Ferretti L, Giardini O. Effect of 3- vs 10-day treatment of urinary tract infections. *J Pediatr* 1984;104:483–484.
7. Madrigal G, Odio CM, Mohs E, Guevara J, McCracken Jr GH. Single dose antibiotic therapy is not as effective as conventional regimens for management of acute urinary tract infections in children. *Pediatr Infect Dis J* 1988;7:316–319.
8. Moffatt M, Embree J, Grimm P, Law B. Short-course antibiotic therapy for urinary tract infections in children. *Am J Dis Child* 1988;142:57–61.
9. Baraff LJ, Bass JW, Fleisher GR, Klein JO, McCracken Jr GH, Powell KR, Schriger DL. Practice guideline for the management of infants and children 0 to 36 months of age with fever without source. *Pediatrics* 1993;92:1–12.
10. Dacher JN, Mandell J, Lebowitz RL. Urinary tract infection in infants in spite of prenatal diagnosis of hydronephrosis. *Pediatr Radiol* 1992;22:401–405.
11. Frenkel LD, and the Multicenter Ceftriaxone Pediatric Study Group. Once-daily administration of ceftriaxone for the treatment of selected serious bacterial infections in children. *Pediatrics* 1988;82:486–491.
12. Bradley JS, Ching DK, Phillips SE. Outpatient therapy of serious pediatric infections with ceftriaxone. *Pediatr Infect Dis J* 1988;7:160–164.
13. Baskin MN, O'Rourke EJ, Fleisher GR. Outpatient treatment of febrile infants 28 to 89 days of age with intramuscular administration of ceftriaxone. *J Pediatr* 1992;120:22–27.
14. Bertino Jr JS, Hayward CJ, Kohlhepp SJ, Nafziger AN. Bioequivalence and reduced severity and duration of injection pain for intramuscular ceftriaxone when administered using buffered lidocaine as a diluent versus 1% lidocaine or water (abst). *Abstracts of the Interscience Conference on Antimicrobial Agents and Chemotherapy.* xxxx:Interscience Conference on Antibiomicrobial Agents and Chemotherapy, 1994:144.
15. Kline MW. The role of aztreonam in treatment of complicated urinary tract infection in children. *Pediatr Infect Dis J* 1989;8:S113–S116.
16. Moellering RC Jr. Emergence of the enterococcus as a significant pathogen. *Clin Infect Dis* 1992;14:1173–1178.
17. Hall LMC, Duke B, Urwin G, Guiney M. Epidemiology of Enterococcus faecalis urinary tract infection in a teaching hospital in London, United Kingdom. *J Clin Microbiol* 1992;30:1953–1957.
18. Felmingham D, Wilson APR, Quintana AI. Enterococcus species in urinary tract infection. *Clin Infect Dis* 1992;15:295–301.
19. Stamm WE, Hooton TM. Management of urinary tract infections in adults. *N Engl J Med* 1993;329:1328–1334.
20. Hovelius B, Mardh P-A. Staphylococcus saprophyticus as a common cause of urinary tract infections. *Rev Infect Dis* 1984;6:328–337.
21. Ena J, Amador C, Martinez C, Ortiz de la Tabla V. Risk factors for acquisition of urinary tract infections caused by ciprofloxacin resistant Escherichia coli. *J Urol* 1995;153:117–120.
22. Winberg J, Böllgren I, Källenius G, Möllby R, Svenson SB. Clinical pyelonephritis and focal renal scarring. A selected review of pathogenesis, prevention, and prognosis. *Pediatr Clin North Am* 1982;29:801–814.
23. LiPuma JJ, Stull TL, Dasen SE, Pidcock KA, Kaye D, Korzeniowski OM. DNA polymorphisms among Escherichia coli isolated from bacteriuric women. *J Infect Dis* 1989;159:526–532.

24. Mittendorf R, Williams MA, Kass EH. Prevention of preterm delivery and low birth weight associated with asymptomatic bacteriuria. *Clin Infect Dis* 1992;14:927–932.
25. Pedler SJ, Bint AJ. Management of bacteriuria in pregnancy. *Drugs* 1987;33:413–421.
26. Gerstner GJ, Müller G, Nahler G. Amoxicillin in the treatment of asymptomatic bacteriuria in pregnancy: a single dose of 3 g amoxicillin versus a 4-day course of 3 doses 750 mg amoxicillin. *Gynecol Obstet Invest* 1989;27:84–87.
27. Lenke RR, VanDorsten JP, Schifrin BS. Pyelonephritis in pregnancy: a prospective randomized trial to prevent recurrent disease evaluating suppressive therapy with nitrofurantoin and close surveillance. *Am J Obstet Gynecol* 1983;146:953–957.
28. Gratacós E, Torres P-J, Vila J, Alonso PL, Cararach V. Screening and treatment of asymptomatic bacteriuria in pregnancy prevent pyelonephritis. *J Infect Dis* 1994;169:1390–1392.
29. Pfau A, Sacks TG. Effective prophylaxis for recurrent urinary tract infections during pregnancy. *Clin Infect Dis* 1992;14:810–814.
30. Uehling DT. Susceptibility factors in ascending urinary tract infection. In: Holliday, Barrott, Arney, eds.*Pediatric nephrology*. 3rd ed. Baltimore: Williams & Wilkins; 1993:986–993.
31. Smith EM, Elder JS. Double antimicrobial prophylaxis in girls with breakthrough urinary tract infections. *Urology* 1994;43:708–713.
32. Majd M, Rushton HG, Jantausch B, Wiedermann BL. Relationship among vesicoureteral reflux, P-fimbriated Escherichia coli, and acute pyelonephritis in children with febrile urinary tract infection. *J Pediatr* 1991;119:578–585.
33. Uehling DT, Vlach RE, Pauli RM, Friedman AL. Vesicourteric reflux in sibships. *Br J Urol* 1992;69:534–537.
34. Page CP, Bohnen JMA, Fletcher JR, McManus AT, Solomkin JS, Wittmann DH. Antimicrobial prophylaxis for surgical wounds. Guidelines for clinical care.*Arch Surg* 1993;128:79–88.
35. Ludwig KA, Carlson MA, Condon RE. Prophylactic antibiotics in surgery. *Annu Rev Med* 1993;44:385–393.
36. Classen DC, Evans RS, Pestotnik SL, Horn SD, Menlove RL, Burke JP. The timing of prophylactic administration of antibiotics and the risk of surgical-wound infection. *N Engl J Med* 1992;326:281–286.
37. Scherz HC, Parsons CL. Prophylactic antibiotics in urology. *Urol Clin North Am* 1987;14:265–271.
38. Waples MJ, Belzer FO, Uehling DT. Living donor nephrectomy: a twenty-year experience. *Urology* 1995;45:207–210.
39. Fowler Jr JE, Perkins T. Presentation, diagnosis and treatment of renal abscesses: 1972–1988. *J Urol* 1994;151:847–851.
40. Brook I. The role of anaerobic bacteria in perinephric and renal abscesses in children. *Pediatrics* 1994;93:261–264.
41. Smellie JM, Poulton A, Prescod NP. Retrospective study of children with renal scarring associated with reflux and urinary infection. *Br Med J* 1994;308:1193–1196.
42. Boscia JA, Abrutyn E, Kaye D. Asymptomatic bacteriuria in elderly persons: treat or do not treat? *Ann Int Med* 1987;106:764–766.
43. Nicolle LE, Mayhew WJ, Bryan L. Prospective randomized comparison of therapy and no therapy for asymptomatic bacteriuria in institutionalized elderly women. *Am J Med* 1987;83:27–33.
44. Nordenstam GR, Brandberg CA, Odén AS, Svanborg Edén CM, Svanborg A. Bacteriuria and mortality in an elderly population. *New Engl J Med* 1986;314:1152–1156.
45. Anderson RU. Prophylaxis of bacteriuria during intermittent catheterization of the acute neurogenic bladder. *J Urol* 1980;123:364–366.
46. Mohler JL, Cowen DL, Flanigan RC. Suppression and treatment of urinary tract infection in patients with an intermittently catheterized neurogenic bladder. *J Urol* 1987;138:336–340.
47. Bakke A, Vollset SE. Risk factors for bacteriuria and clinical urinary tract infection in patients treated with clean intermittent catheterization. *J Urol* 1993;149:527–531.
48. Waller L, Jonsson O, Norlèn L, Sullivan L. Clean intermittent catheterization in spinal cord injury patients: long-term followup of a hydrophilic low friction technique. *J Urol* 1995;153:345–348.
49. Chawla JC, Stickler DJ, Clayton CL. Some observations on urinary tract infections in patients undergoing long-term catheterization. *J Hosp Infect* 1982;3:39–47.

50. Stamm WE. Catheter-associated urinary tract infections: epidemiology, pathogenesis, and prevention. *Am J Med* 1991;91 (Suppl):S65–S71.
51. Britt MR, Garibaldi RA, Miller WA, Hebertson RM, Burke JP. Antimicrobial prophylaxis for catheter-associated bacteriuria. *Antimicrob Agents Chemother* 1977;11:240–243.
52. Van Der Wall E, Verkooyen RP, Mintjes-De Groot J, Oostinga J, Van Dijk A, Hustinx WNM, Verbrugh HA. Prophylactic ciprofloxacin for catheter-associated urinary tract infection. *Lancet* 1992;339:946–951.
53. Ried G, Denstedt JD, Kang YS, Lam D, Nause C. Microbial adhesion and biofilm formation on ureteral stents in vitro and in vivo. *J Urol* 1992;148:1592–1594.
54. Ohkawa M, Sugata T, Sawaki M, Nakashima T, Fuse H, Hisazumi H. Bacterial and crystal adherence to the surfaces of indwelling urethral catheters. *J Urol* 1990;143:717–721.
55. Reid G, Kang YS, Lacerte M, Tieszer C, Hayes KC. Bacterial biofilm formation on the bladder epithelium of spinal cord injured patients. II. Toxic outcome on cell viability. *Paraplegia* 1993;31:494–499.
56. Reid G. Do antibiotics clear bladder infections? *J Urol* 1994;152:865–867.
57. Fowler JE. Bacteriology of branched renal calculi and accompanying urinary tract infection. *J Urol* 1984;131:213–215.
58. Lerner SP, Gleeson MJ, Griffith DP. Infection stones. *J Urol* 141:753–759.
59. Grenabo L, Hedelin H, Pettersson S. Urinary infection stones caused by Ureaplasma urealyticum: a review. *Scand J Infect Dis* 1988;53:46–49.
60. Hedelin H, Brorson J-E, Grenabo L, Pettersson S. Ureaplasma urealyticum and upper urinary tract stones. *Br J Urol* 1984;56:244–249.
61. Rose GA, Rosenbaum TP. Recurrent infection stones with apparently negative cultures. The case for blind antibacterial treatment. *Br J Urol* 1992;69:234–239.
62. Ohkawa M, Tokunaga S, Nakashima T, Yamaguchi K, Orito M, Hisazumi H. Composition of urinary calculi related to urinary tract infection. *J Urol* 1992;148:995–997.
63. Beck EM, Riehle RA Jr. The fate of residual fragments after extracorporeal shock wave lithotripsy monotherapy of infection stones. *J Urol* 1991;145:6–10.
64. Michaels EK, Fowler JE Jr, Mariano M. Bacteriuria following extracorporeal shock wave lithotripsy of infection stones. *J Urol* 1988;140:254–256.
65. Ramadan MA, Tawfik AF, El-Kersh TA, Shibl AM. In vitro activity of subinhibitory concentrations of quinolones on urea-splitting bacteria: effect on urease activity and on cell surface hydrophobicity. *J Infect Dis* 1995;171:483–486.
66. Meares EM Jr. Prostatitis: review of pharmacokinetics and therapy. *Rev Infect Dis* 1982;4:475–483.
67. Naber KG. Use of quinolones in urinary tract infections and prostatitis. *Rev Infect Dis* 1989;11:S1321–S1337.
68. Boerema JBJ, Dalhoff A, Debruyne FMY. Ciprofloxacin distribution in prostatic tissue and fluid following oral administration. *Chemotherapy* 1985;31:13–18.
69. Bergeron MG, Thabet M, Roy R, Lessard C, Foucault P. Norfloxacin penetration into human renal and prostatic tissues. *Antimicrob Agents Chemother* 1985;28:349–350.
70. Nielsen OS, Maigaard S, Frimodt-Moller N, Madsen PO. Prophylactic antibiotics in transurethral prostatectomy. *J Urol* 1981;126:60–62.
71. Madsen PO. Editorial: antibacterial therapy and prophylaxis in transurethral surgery. *Urol Res* 1986;14:177–178.
72. Prokocimer P, Quazza M, Gibert C, Lemoine JE, Joly ML, Dureuil B, Moulonguet A, Manuel C, Desmonts JM. Short-term prophylactic antibiotics in patients undergoing prostatectomy: report of a double-blind randomized trial with 2 intravenous doses of cefotaxime. *J Urol* 1986;135:60–64.
73. Viitanen J, Talja M, Jussila E, Nurmi M, Permi J, Puolakka V-M, Rintala E, Salmela H, Tiitinen J, Tuhkanen K, Elo J. Randomized controlled study of chemoprophylaxis in transurethral prostatectomy. *J Urol* 1993;150:1715–1717.
74. Desai KM, Abrams PH, White LO. A double-blind comparative trial of short-term orally administered enoxacin in the prevention of urinary infection after elective transurethral prostatectomy: a clinical and pharmacokinetic study. *J Urol* 1988;139:1232–1234.
75. Crawford ED, Berger NS, Davis MA, Donohue RE. Prevention of urinary tract infection and bacteremia following transurethral surgery: oral lomefloxacin compared to parenteral cefotaxime. *J Urol* 1992;147:1053–1055.

76. Thompson PM, Pryor JP, Williams JP, Eyers DE, Dulake C, Scully MF, Kakkar VV. The problem of infection after prostatic biopsy: the case for the transperineal approach. *Br J Urol* 1982;54:736–740.
77. Roach MB, Figueroa TE, McBride D, George WJ, Neal Jr DE. Ciprofloxacin versus gentamicin in prophylaxis against bacteremia in transrectal prostate needle biopsy. *Urology* 1991;38:84–87.
78. Goldwasser B, Bogokowsky B, Nativ O, Sidi AA, Jonas P, Many M. Prophylactic antimicrobial treatment in transurethral prostatectomy. *Urology* 1983;22:136–138.
79. Desmond PM, Clark J, Thompson IM, Zeidman EJ, Mueller EJ. Morbidity with contemporary prostate biopsy. *J Urol* 1993;150:1425–1426.
80. Aus G, Hermansson CG, Hugosson J, Pedersen KV. Transrectal ultrasound examination of the prostate: complications and acceptance by patients. *Br J Urol* 1993;71:457–459.
81. Collins GN, Lloyd SN, Hehir M, McKelvie GB. Multiple transrectal ultrasound-guided prostatic biopsies—true morbidity and patient acceptance. *Br J Urol* 1993;71:460–463.
82. Vallancien G, Prapotnich D, Veillon B, Brisset JM, Andre-Bougaran J. Systematic prostatic biopsies in 100 men with no suspicion of cancer on digital rectal examination. *J Urol* 1991;146:1308–1312.

Antibiotic Therapy in Urology,
edited by S. Grant Mulholland, M.D.,
Lippincott-Raven Publishers, Philadelphia © 1996.

Chapter 11

Antimicrobial Therapy in the Management of Infected Renal Calculi

Jackson E. Fowler, Jr.

Division of Urology, University of Mississippi Medical Center, Jackson, Mississippi 39216

Approximately 5% of renal calculi are composed of magnesium ammonium phosphate (struvite) and carbonate apatite, and are colonized by bacteria. These "infection stones" are usually large, cause obstruction of the intrarenal collecting system, and may lead to bacterial nephritis or intrarenal and perirenal abscess formation. If they are left untreated, the incidence of death from renal failure or sepsis approaches 30% (1,2).

Infected renal calculi are seen primarily in women and are remarkably infrequent in children. However, they may develop in patients of either sex and any age who have chronically infected urine resulting from urinary diversion or exteriorized catheters. Infection stones are the most common cause of persistent bacteriuria in women and probably follow chronic bacterial prostatitis as the second most common cause of persistent bacteriuria in men.

The treatment of infected renal calculi has changed substantially with the advent of percutaneous nephrostolithotomy and extracorporeal shock wave lithotripsy (ESWL). However, the basic principles of diagnosis and management established when open surgery was the only available intervention remain the same.

ETIOLOGY AND PATHOGENESIS

Metabolic disorders that predispose to urinary calculogenesis have no role in the pathogenesis of infection stones. Rather, the stones result from infection of the urine by bacteria that synthesize the enzyme urease (2,3,4,5) (Fig. 1). Ammonium is released by the breakdown of urea by urease, the urine becomes highly alkaline, and struvite and carbonate

- **bacteriuria caused by an organism that synthesizes the enzyme urease**
- **urinary urea $\xrightarrow{\text{urease}}$ NH_4 and OH**
- **urinary pH increases to 8 - 10**
- **$MgNH_4PO_4$ (struvite) and Ca_{10} $(PO_4)CO_3$ (carbonate apatite) precipitate**
- **infecting bacteria incorporated into developing stone**
- **antimicrobials incapable of eradicating bacteria within stone**

FIG. 1. Pathogenesis of infection stones. (From Fowler, ref. 18, with permission.)

apatite crystallize (6). Stone growth is characteristically rapid, and most appear as "staghorns" occupying the renal pelvis and one or more infundibula and calyces when discovered. Incorporation of the infecting bacteria within the stone creates a focus of infection that is generally resistant to antimicrobial therapy and results in persistent bacteriuria (4,5,7).

A technique for culture of urinary stones devised by Nemoy and Stamey (5) has done much to clarify the role of infection in the process of calculogenesis. The cultures also have clinical value because antimicrobial therapy following the treatment of struvite calculi is most reasonably guided by the susceptibilities of the organism or organisms that colonize the stone. The culture methods are designed to distinguish bacteria within a stone from surface colonization (Fig. 2). A portion of the stone is washed consecutively in four test tubes containing 5 ml of sterile saline and then crushed in the fourth tube. One-tenth of a milliliter of fluid from washes 1 and 4, and of the fluid of the crushed stone, is quantitatively cultured using routine techniques. An increased density of an isolate in the fluid of the crushed stone compared with the fluid of wash 4 is considered evidence of bacteria within the stone. Usually the density of bacteria in the fluid of a crushed infection stone exceeds that of the fourth wash fluid by 100- to 1,000-fold (Table 1).

Two reports have detailed the spectrum of bacterial species that colonize renal struvite calculi (4,8). In both studies patients had received antimicrobial therapy for varying periods before stone removal, all of the stones were extracted by open surgery, and all of the isolates were localized to the substance of the calculi. Bacteria capable of urease synthesis were isolated from 77% and 90% of the calculi, and 71% and

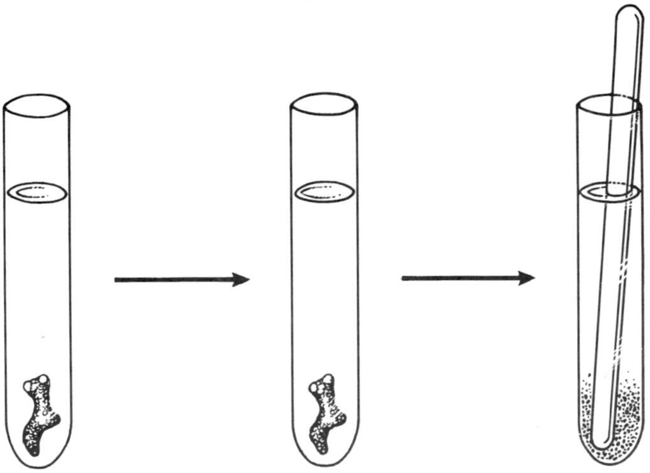

FIG. 2. Culture technique for localization of bacteria to substance of a calculus. (From Fowler, ref. 18, with permission.)

86% of the urease-positive isolates were *Proteus mirabilis*. The predominance of *P. mirabilis* is consistent with observations that the urease of *P. mirabilis* hydrolyzes urea at rates 6 to 25 times faster than the ureases of other bacterial species (9).

In some instances yeasts or bacteria that do not synthesize urease were isolated alone or in combination with *P. mirabilis*. Any organism that infects the urine during the precipitation of struvite, therefore, may become incorporated within the developing stone. Finally, a small pro-

Table 1. *Organisms localized to renal struvite calculi*

		Bacteria		
Number	Organism	Wash fluid 1	Wash fluid 4	Crushed stone fluid
1	*P. mirabilis*	800	300	4,600
2	*P. mirabilis*	260	120	15,000
3	*P. mirabilis*	200	140	2,100
4	*P. mirabilis*	120	20	20,000
5	*P. aeruginosa*	100,000	39,000	100,000
6	*P. mirabilis*	0	0	370
7	*P. mirabilis*	60	20	7,000
8	*P. mirabilis*	0	0	4,300

From Fowler, ref. 4.

Table 2. *Organisms localized to renal struvite calculi*

Organism	Thompson and Stamey, No. (%)	Fowler, No. (%)
P. mirabilis	21 (43)	9 (41)
K. pneumoniae	2 (4)	2 (9)
P. aeruginosa	1 (2)	2 (9)
S. marcescens	-	1
S. aureus	2 (4)	-
E. coli[a]	2 (4)	-
Yeast[a]	1 (2)	-
P. mirabilis plus other isolate	17 (35)	3 (14)
P. rettgeri plus other isolate	1 (2)	-
Sterile	2 (4)	5 (23)
Total	49	22

From Thompson and Stamey, ref. 8, and Fowler, ref. 4.
[a]Organism not capable of urease synthesis.

portion of the calculi were sterile. This suggests that struvite may precipitate in the absence of infection, or that antimicrobial therapy may occasionally sterilize a developing stone. There is also evidence that infection of the urine with *Ureaplasma urealyticum*, a urease-producing mycoplasma organism that is not detectable with routine culture techniques, may cause struvite renal calculi (10,11).

DIAGNOSIS

Sequential urinary tract infections caused by an organism capable of urease synthesis are the hallmarks of infection stones. Generally speaking, the urine can be sterilized with appropriate antimicrobial therapy, but bacteriuria occurs promptly after treatment. Interestingly, the magnitude of irritative voiding symptoms in patients with infection stones and persistent *P. mirabilis* bacteriuria is often minimal. This may account in part for the large size of infected calculi at diagnosis.

Most infection stones are visible on plain radiographs of the abdomen. The degree of calcification, however, is variable, and some stones are seen only with plain-film tomograms. All infection stones are identifiable with unenhanced computed tomography. Such imaging may be rewarding in the evaluation of persistent bacteriuria from an indeterminate site that is caused by an organism capable of urease synthesis, or for the identification of residual stone particles in patients with persistent bacteriuria following interventional treatments. The relative sensitivities of the abdominal radiograph and unenhanced computed tomography for the detection of minimally calcified infection stones are demonstrated in Fig. 3.

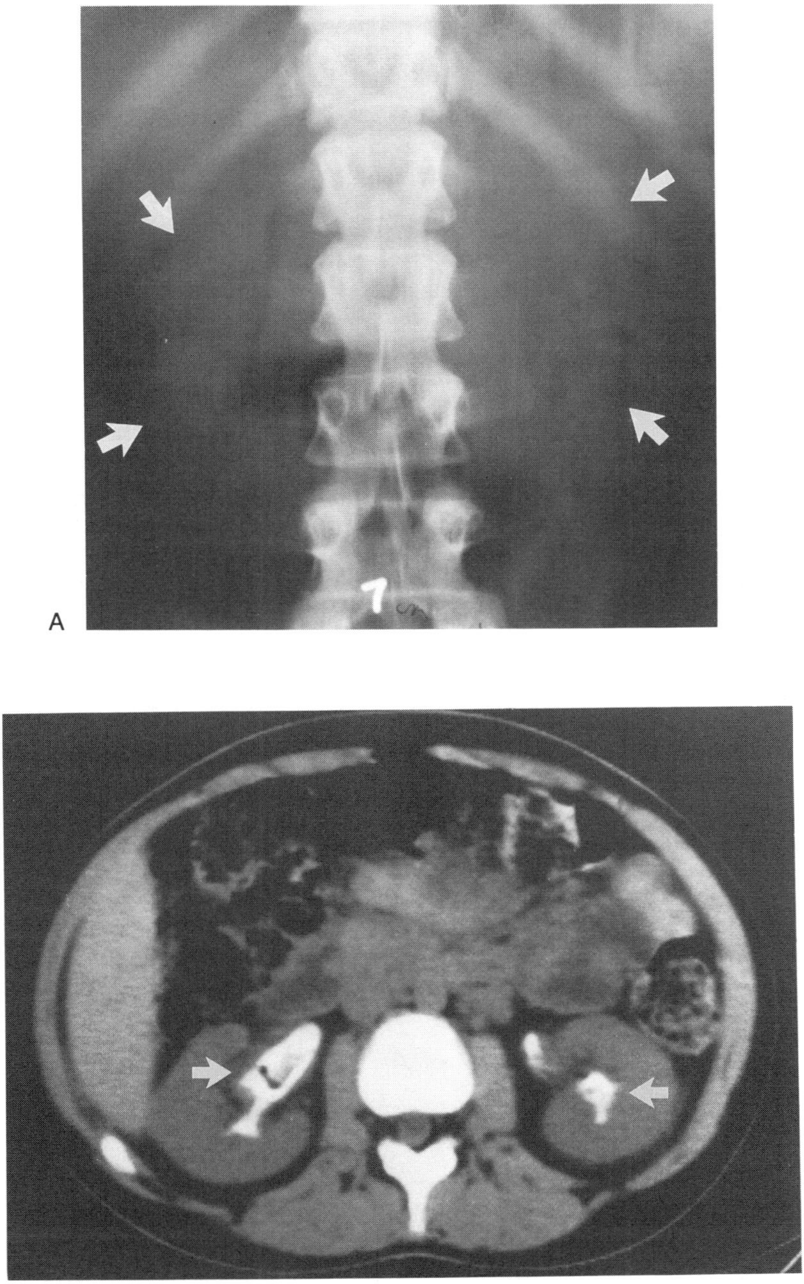

A

B

FIG. 3. Abdominal radiograph (**A**) and unenhanced computed tomogram (**B**) of minimally calcified bilateral branched struvite calculi. (From Fowler, ref. 18, with permission.)

ANTIMICROBIAL THERAPY FOR BACTERIURIA: GENERAL CONSIDERATIONS

Antimicrobial Concentrations in the Urine

The targets of antimicrobials for the treatment of bacteriuria are microorganisms within the urine, and the antibacterial activity of most drugs is related to their concentration at the site of infection. It reasonably follows that therapeutic success or failure is a function of drug activity at levels achievable in the urine rather than at concentrations achievable in the serum. This concept is of substantial clinical relevance because most antimicrobials are physiologically concentrated by the kidneys. The approximate relationship between urinary and serum levels of oral antimicrobials used commonly for the treatment of bacteriuria is shown in Table 3. Note that the urinary concentrations of most of the agents listed are 50 to 200 times greater than the serum concentrations.

Several fundamental considerations support the importance of urinary antibiotic concentrations in the treatment of bacteriuria. First, nitrofurantoin, nalidixic acid, and cinoxacin are effective for the treatment of many urinary tract infections but are not active against gram-negative bacilli at serum concentrations. Second, several clinical investigations have shown that infections caused by organisms judged resistant to an administered drug by the Kirby-Bauer assay (which tests susceptibility to antimicrobials at concentrations achievable in the serum) can be eradicated with the apparently inactive agent (12–17).

Table 3. *Approximate ratio of urine and serum concentrations of selected oral antimicrobial agents*[a]

Agent	Urine/Serum
Ampicillin	100
Carbenicillin[b]	75
Cephalexin	150
Cinoxacin[b]	200
Ciprofloxacin	300
Nalidixic acid[b]	3
Nitrofurantoin[b]	100
Norfloxacin	300
Penicillin G	300
Sulfonamides	3
Tetracycline	250
Trimethoprim	100

From Fowler, ref. 18, with permission.
[a]At recommended dosage in adults with normal renal function.
[b]Therapeutic concentrations not achievable in serum.

The reader should note, however, that serum rather than urine drug levels are of therapeutic importance when bacteriuria is accompanied by infection of the kidney or other soft tissues. Invasive infections are unlikely to respond to treatment if the serum drug concentration is subtherapeutic.

Treatment Regimens for Bacteriuria

Antimicrobial therapy in the management of bacteriuria is properly characterized as curative, prophylactic, or suppressive (18).

Curative therapy is intended to eradicate an existing infection and to restore the urinary system to its normal sterile physiologic state. Curative therapy usually consists of 3 to 5 days of treatment with an antibiotic that is administered at conventional doses. By definition, persistent infections, such as those associated with infected renal calculi, are usually refractory to curative treatment regimens.

Prophylactic therapy is designed to prevent urinary reinfection by the long-term administration of antimicrobials at low doses and is usually employed in women who are highly susceptible to urinary reinfections. The antimicrobial agents used for prophylactic therapy parallel those that are utilized for suppressive therapy.

Suppressive therapy is used in the management of persistent infections to suppress or eliminate bacterial growth in the urine. Sterilization of the infected focus within the urinary system, such as an infected renal stone, is not a realistic or intended therapeutic goal. The selection of an appropriate drug for suppressive therapy is dictated by antimicrobial susceptibility testing and the likelihood that an active agent will be well tolerated during long term and, possibly, indefinite administration. Quantitative susceptibility testing that estimates the activity of antibiotics against the infecting organism at concentrations achievable in the urine may be necessary to identify the most appropriate agent. Nitrofurantoin, trimethoprim/sulfamethoxazole, trimethoprim, or a fluoroquinolone antibiotic are excellent agents for susceptible infections because of the relative infrequency of adverse effects during long-term therapy. The drugs are usually administered once daily at about 25% of the recommended dose.

ANTIMICROBIAL THERAPY FOR INFECTION STONES

Antimicrobial therapy for infection stones is always suppressive, but the clinical circumstances dictate drug selection and dosage.

Antibiotic Therapy After Diagnosis

Some patients with infection stones present with symptomatic pyelonephritis or with an intrarenal or perinephric abscess. For example, in a recent study of 61 patients with renal abscesses, 18% had associated renal stones, and the vast majority of the calculi had a branched appearance consistent with an infection stone (19). In these situations, treatment of the parenchymal infection or abscess, or of co-existing renal obstruction, takes precedence over treatment of the stone. The appropriate management of such potentially lethal conditions is addressed in other chapters of this book.

In patients with bacteriuria only at the time of diagnosis, the urine should be sterilized with an appropriate oral antibiotic given at conventional doses for 5 to 7 days. Suppressive therapy is then instituted to maintain a sterile urine until the stone is removed by open surgery, percutaneous nephrostolithotomy, ESWL, or combined therapy with percutaneous nephrostolithotomy and ESWL.

Perioperative Antibiotic Therapy

Invasive or extracorporeal treatments for infection stones should be considered as "contaminated" procedures since some degree of bacterial colonization of the stone surface should be anticipated and because bacteria are inevitably liberated from the substance of the stone during fragmentation. For these reasons, and because anesthesia is required for the procedures, the patient should receive parenteral antibiotics at full dosage in the perioperative period.

Posttreatment Antimicrobial Therapy

Minute flecks of stone material adhere to the mucosa of the intrarenal collecting system after successful removal of an infection stone by any technique, and there is convincing clinical evidence that antimicrobial therapy may sterilize small stone particles (20). To exploit the latter possibility, treatment with an appropriate antibiotic at full oral dosage for 2 to 4 weeks after the intervention is advisable.

Serial urine cultures are obtained after the posttreatment antibiotic therapy has been discontinued to determine whether the urinary tract has been sterilized and whether further antimicrobial therapy is warranted. A urine culture should be obtained every month for 6 months and then every 6 months for a minimum of 2 years. As a general rule, isolation of the same organism that was recovered from the urine before treatment, or that was recovered from the substance of the stone, is unequivocable evidence of a residual infected stone fragment or, rarely, persistent infection of focally ischemic renal parenchyma. This occurrence mandates the resumption of suppressive antimicrobial therapy to prevent formation of another infection stone.

Antimicrobial Therapy with Persistent Stone Fragments After ESWL

Incomplete stone removal after open lithotomy or percutaneous nephrostolithotomy for struvite renal calculi is often associated with perpetuation of pre-existing persistent bacteriuria and stone recurrence (1,21–23). This phenomenon has raised concerns about the efficacy of ESWL for the treatment of struvite renal calculi since 30–40% of affected patients who are treated with ESWL alone have radiographically identifiable stone particles in the renal collecting system for 1 year after treatment (23,24).

Dr. Eli Michaels and I, however, have demonstrated that the particles of struvite renal calculi that pass spontaneously after ESWL are usually sterile (20). This appears to reflect a susceptibility of finely pulverized stone material to sterilization with antibiotics that are delivered in the perioperative period and suggests that retained stone particles after ESWL do not increase the risk for persistent bacteriuria or stone recurrence.

To investigate the latter possibility, Dr. Michaels and I prospectively studied 22 otherwise healthy women who had struvite renal stones and persistent *P. mirabilis* bacteriuria before ESWL (25). Each received parenteral gentamicin in the perioperative period and full-dose trimethoprim/sulfamethoxazole or trimethoprim for 2 weeks after treatment and, if applicable, for 2 weeks following the removal of ureteral stents or nephrostomy drainage tubes. The patients were followed for 16 to 52 months (mean, 39 months) after ESWL with frequent urine cultures and plain abdominal radiographs.

Nineteen of the 22 patients (86%) were cured of the persistent bacteriuria. Of these 19 patients, 16 had retained stone particles after treatment and 10 had retained stone particles at the last follow-up. One of the patients who was rendered stone-free had a *P. mirabilis* reinfection at 20 months after treatment and developed a new stone.

Three of the patients (14%) had continued persistent *P. mirabilis* bacteriuria after discontinuing the antibiotics, although one was subsequently cured of the infection with prolonged suppressive antimicrobial therapy and extraction of a new ureteral stone. The remaining patient had expansion of retained stone particles after 51 months of intermittent antibiotic therapy.

This prospective study showed that ESWL and a relatively short course of antimicrobial therapy usually eradicate the persistent bacteriuria that accompanies infection stones and that sterile stone particles do not enlarge during the first 2 to 4 years after treatment. However, the results also demonstrated that a stone-free kidney is an unrealistic objective of ESWL for struvite renal calculi and emphasize the concept that the urinary bacteriology rather than the presence of persistent stone fragments is the most important parameter for determining the necessity of further therapeutic intervention or long-term suppressive antimicrobial therapy.

Antimicrobial Therapy During Renal Irrigation

Hemiacidrin (Renacidin) is a mixture of water-soluble multivalent organic acids that dissolve struvite and calcium apatite (26). Hemiacidrin irrigation of the renal collecting system has been employed as primary treatment for infected renal calculi (27) and for the dissolution of identifiable or suspected residual stone fragments after nephrolithotomy or ESWL (28–33). The irrigant is generally delivered through a nephrostomy tube as shown in Fig. 4, and a variety of precautions are necessary to prevent flank pain, urothelial inflammation, or increased serum magnesium levels (18). Acute bacterial nephritis can develop during irrigation and is potentiated by persistent elevation of the intrarenal pressure above 15 cm H_2O. To prevent infectious complications, a urine specimen that is aspirated from the nephrostomy tube is cultured on a daily basis and an aminoglycoside or fluoroquinolone antibiotic is administered throughout the period of irrigation.

Colonization of the urine with *Candida albicans* is not infrequent during prolonged renal irrigations. The risks of candiduria appear to be minimal if the infusion pressure is low and the patient is not febrile. The fungal infection usually resolves spontaneously when the irrigation is completed, and antifungal therapy is not indicated in the absence of clinical evidence of candidemia.

Primary Antimicrobial Therapy for Infection Stones

On occasion the physician encounters a debilitated patient with an infection stone who is not an acceptable candidate for percutaneous nephrolithotomy or ESWL. We have managed several such patients with long-term suppressive antimicrobial therapy using a fluoroquinolone antibiotic and have maintained a sterile urine for as long as 4 years. As would be anticipated, stone enlargement has not been observed because

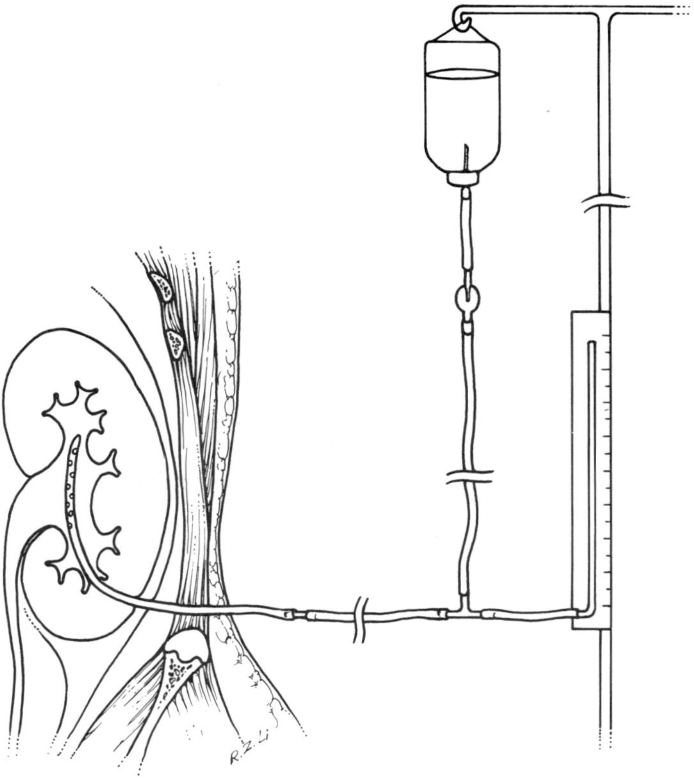

FIG. 4. Technique for hemiacidrin irrigation of the renal collecting system. (From Fowler, ref. 18, with permission.)

there is no bacteriuria to produce a highly alkaline urine. None of the patients have experienced fever or clinically significant flank pain during treatment.

Primary antimicrobial therapy does not lead to stone dissolution, and catastrophic infectious complications are possible if the patient is noncompliant. Nonetheless, this therapeutic approach may be the only alternative in some cases.

CASE REPORTS

The following case reports illustrate the principles of management of infection stones elaborated above.

Case 1: *Staphylococcus saprophyticus* as a Cause of Infected Urinary Calculus

A 31-year-old pregnant woman had the acute onset of dysuria and frequency in March 1982. *Staphylococcus* was isolated from a voided urine specimen (Table 4). Oral ampicillin therapy was begun on March 19, but hospitalization was required on March 21 because of fever, chills, and left flank pain. The urine culture on admission showed $>10^4$ bacteria per milliliter that were not characterized. The patient responded promptly to 2 days of treatment with intravenous ampicillin and then received oral ampicillin for 8 additional days.

During the remainder of her pregnancy she had intermittent back pain and irritative voiding symptoms but no further febrile episodes. There was persistent staphylococcal bacteriuria despite a 10-day course of oral ampicillin starting on June 23 and a 16-day course starting on July 30. The infecting organisms were uniformly susceptible in vitro to ampicillin. A healthy child with an estimated gestational age of 37 weeks was delivered on August 13.

The patient was not seen again until December 14, 1983, when she developed fever and left upper quadrant pain. During the intervening 16 months she had had urinary frequency and dysuria but sought no medical attention. An ampicillin-sensitive *S. saprophyticus* was isolated from the voided urine specimen. Dilatation of the left renal pelvis and upper ureter was seen on ultrasonographic examination, and a plain radiograph of the abdomen showed a 2- by 1-cm calcification in the left

Table 4. *Urinary bacteriology and treatment of woman with infection stone caused by* S. saprophyticus *(case 1)*

		Urine culture	
Date	Antimicrobial therapy (days on or off)	Organisms	Bacteria/ml
12 Mar 1982	First visit	Staphylococci	$>10^5$
21 Mar 1982	Ampicillin (2 on)	Sterile	
12 Apr 1982	Ampicillin (12 off)	Staphylococci	10^4
23 Jun 1982	Ampicillin (41 off)	Sterile	
29 Jun 1982	Ampicillin (6 on)	Sterile	
30 Jul 1982	Ampicillin (27 off)	Staphylococci	10^4
06 Aug 1982	Ampicillin (7 on)	Staphylococci	10^5
13 Aug 1982	Ampicillin (14 on)	Staphylococci	$>10^5$
14 Dec 1983		*S. saprophyticus*	$>10^5$
16 Dec 1983	Ampicillin (2 on)	Ureterolithotomy	
20 Dec 1983	Ampicillin (6 on)	Sterile	
12 Jan 1984	TMP/SMX (5 off)	Sterile	
14 Mar 1984	TMP/SMX (67 off)	Sterile	

TMP/SMX, trimethoprim/sulfamethoxazole.
From Fowler, ref. 36.

lower quadrant (Fig. 5a). This was demonstrated to be a partially obstructive ureteral calculus with an intravenous pyelogram (Fig. 5b). Intravenous ampicillin therapy was instituted and a left ureterolithotomy was done on the third hospital day.

Culture of the stone revealed *S. saprophyticus* bacteria in the following densities: wash fluid 1, 100/ml; wash fluid 4, 20/ml; crushed stone fluid, 480/ml. Approximately 52% of the calculus was composed of struvite and approximately 38% was composed of carbonate apatite.

The intravenous ampicillin therapy was continued for 4 days after surgery. The patient was then treated with trimethoprim/sulfamethoxazole until January 7, 1984. Voided urine specimens obtained 5 and 67 days later were sterile.

Comment

To my knowledge this is the only well-documented case of an infected struvite calculus caused by *S. saprophyticus* and resulting in persistent *S. saprophyticus* bacteriuria. Three patients with persistent *S. saprophyticus* bacteriuria who had co-existing renal calculi have been reported (34), and one patient with an obstructive ureteral calculus associated with *S. saprophyticus* bacteriuria and bacteremia has been described (35). In these cases, however, the compositions and bacteriology of the stones were not characterized.

This case demonstrates that bacteriuria caused by any organism capable of urease synthesis may result in the precipitation of struvite and the formation of a calculus. *S. saprophyticus*, like most staphylococcal species, synthesizes urease. The case also underscores the concept that all patients with culture-proven persistent bacteriuria require urologic investigation.

Case 2: Bacteriologic Cure After Treatment of Struvite Calculus With ESWL

A 29-year-old woman was referred for lithotripsy in June 1986. She had experienced multiple symptomatic urinary tract infections during the preceding 5 years, but the bacteriology of the infections was not known. Culture of a voided urine specimen revealed *P. mirabilis* (Table 5),and a branched calculus was seen on a plain radiograph of the abdomen (Fig. 6a). She was treated with trimethoprim/sulfamethoxazole at full oral dosage and was begun on parenteral gentamicin after hospital admission on June 22. The following day, a double-coiled right ureteral stent was placed and the stone was partially pulverized with ESWL. The gentamicin therapy was continued during the following week and the remainder of the stone was pulverized with ESWL on June 30.

A 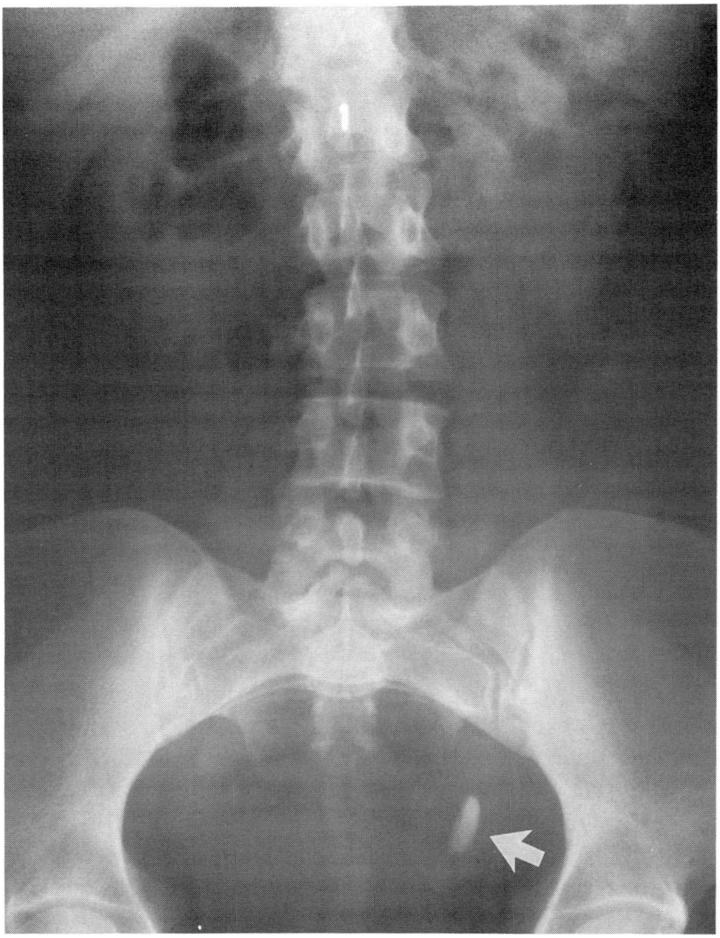

FIG. 5. Radiographs from case report 1. (**A**) Plain radiograph of the abdomen showing distal left ureteral calculus (*arrow*).

Cultures of the wash fluid and crushed stone fluid specimens were all sterile. Approximately 30% of the stone was composed of struvite and approximately 70% was composed of carbonate apatite.

Trimethoprim/sulfamethoxazole at full oral dosage was begun at hospital discharge on July 2. Thirty-three days later, a plain radiograph of the abdomen revealed complete clearance of stone particles in the ureter but the presence of residual particles in the renal pelvis (Fig. 6b). The ureteral stent was removed and trimethoprim/sulfamethoxazole therapy was continued for an additional 2 weeks.

The patient was asymptomatic and the urine remained sterile until December 17, when she developed a symptomatic infection caused by *Citrobacter freundii*. The urine was sterilized with norfloxacin but symptomatic bacteriuria again with *C. freundii* was documented on February 3,

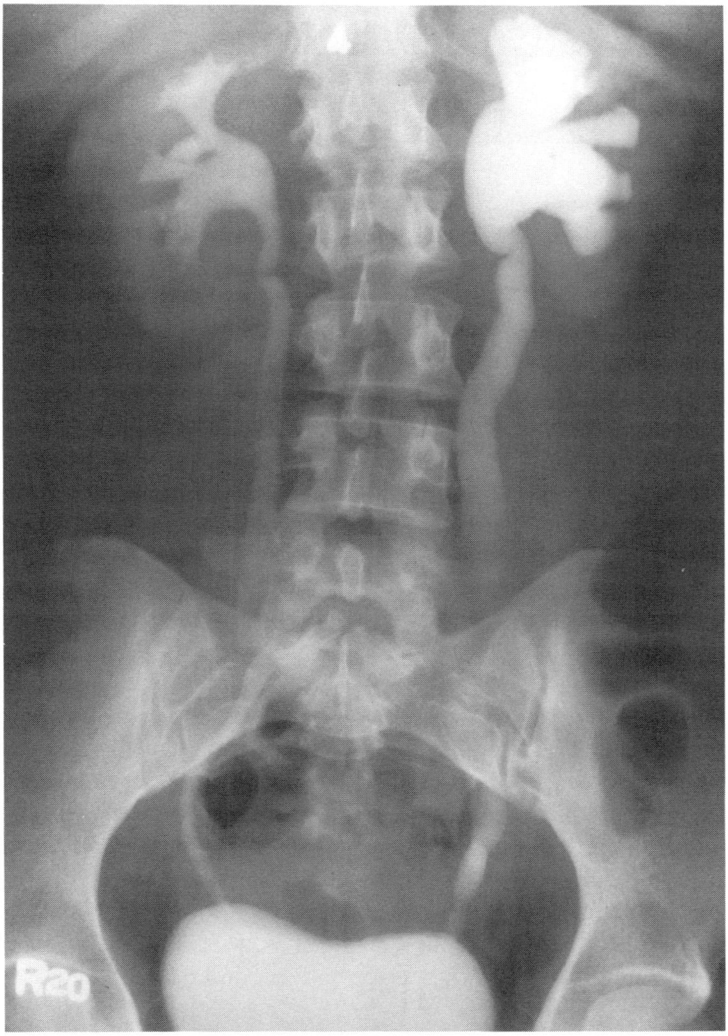

B

FIG. 5. Radiographs from case report 1. (**B**) Intravenous pyelogram showing partial ureteral obstruction. (From Fowler, ref. 18, with permission.)

1987. This infection was treated successfully with norfloxacin, and the urine remained sterile during the ensuing 6 months. The most recent radiograph of the abdomen, obtained in July 1987, revealed persistent stone particles within the renal collecting system (Fig. 6c).

Comment

This case illustrates the primary components of our approach to the treatment of infection stones with ESWL. A sterile urine is maintained

Table 5. *Urinary bacteriology and treatment of woman with P. mirabilis bacteriuria and struvite calculus treated by ESWL (case 2)*

		Urine culture	
Date	Antimicrobial therapy (days on or off)	Organisms	Bacteria/ml
1981–1986	Multiple episodes of symptomatic bacteriuria		
20 Jun 1986	First visit	*P. mirabilis*	>10^5
23 Jun 1986	TMP/SMX (3 on)	Ureteral stent and ESWL	
30 Jun 1986	Gentamicin (7 on)	ESWL	
02 Jul 1986	Gentamicin (9 on)	Sterile	
04 Aug 1986	TMP/SMX (33 on)	Stent removed	
18 Aug 1986	TMP/SMX (47 on)	Sterile	
29 Aug 1986	TMP/SMX (11 off)	Sterile	
16 Sept 1986	TMP/SMX (29 off)	Sterile	
04 Nov 1986	TMP/SMX (78 off)	Sterile	
17 Dec 1986	TMP/SMX (121 off)	*C. freundii*	10^4
27 Dec 1986	NFX (10 on)	Sterile	
03 Feb 1987	NFX (28 off)	*C. freundii*	10^4
16 Feb 1987	NFX (2 off)	Sterile	
06 Jul 1987	NFX (200 off)	Sterile	

From Fowler, ref. 18.
TMP/SMX, trimethoprim/sulfamethoxazole; NFX, norfloxacin.

before treatment with suppressive antimicrobial therapy and a parental antibiotic is administered before treatment. A double-coiled ureteral stent is positioned if technically possible. After complete pulverization of the stone, oral antimicrobial therapy is administered to reduce the risks of obstructive bacterial nephritis. The ureteral stent is not removed until all ureteral fragments have cleared. Antimicrobials are then administered for 2 additional weeks after stent removal. The patient is then monitored with monthly urine cultures and plain abdominal radiographs.

In this case residual stone particles have persisted in the renal collecting system for a year following ESWL. The particles have not enlarged, nor has there been culture evidence of persistent *P. mirabilis* bacteriuria. The patient developed a symptomatic urinary reinfection caused by *C. freundii* that was ultimately eradicated with antimicrobial therapy. For reasons that are unclear, a urine culture was not obtained after the completion of the initial course of norfloxacin, but we believe that the second episode of *C. freundii* bacteriuria reflected inadequate treatment of the first infection.

As demonstrated in this case, women with infected renal calculi may be susceptible to urinary reinfection. For this reason meaningful conclusions about the impact of ESWL, or any treatment for infected renal calculi, on persistent bacteriuria must necessarily be based on knowledge of the bacterial species responsible for the infections before and after treatment.

Case 3: Persistent Bacteriuria After Treatment of Struvite Calculus With ESWL

A 56-year-old woman was referred for lithotripsy in January 1986. She had experienced intermittent dysuria and frequency for 2 months before presentation but had no history of bacteriuria. Culture of a voided urine specimen revealed *P. mirabilis* (Table 6), and a branched calculus in the right kidney was seen on the plain radiograph of the abdomen (Fig. 7a).

She was treated with trimethoprim at full oral dosage for 7 days before ESWL and with gentamicin after hospital admission on February 3. A double-coiled ureteral stent could not be maneuvered into the right renal pelvis, and the stone was pulverized without the benefit of ancillary drainage procedures. Gentamicin therapy was continued for 2 days after ESWL and the patient was discharged 3 days after treatment.

Culture of the wash fluids and crushed stone fluid revealed *P. mirabilis*, but the density of the isolates in the crushed stone fluid culture did not exceed that in the culture of the fourth wash fluid. Approximately 60%

Table 6. *Urinary bacteriology and treatment of woman with P. mirabilis bacteriuria and struvite calculus treated by ESWL (case 1)*

		Urine culture	
Date	Antimicrobial therapy (days on or off)	Organisms	Bacteria/ml
28 Jan 1986	First visit	*P. mirabilis*	$>10^5$
3 Feb 1986	TMP (7 on)	ESWL	
5 Feb 1986	Gentamicin (3 on)	Sterile	
19 Feb 1986	TMP (14 on)	Sterile	
26 Mar 1986	TMP (35 off)	*P. mirabilis*	10^4
21 May 1986	TMP (56 on)	Sterile	
24 Jun 1986	TMP (90 on)	Sterile	
5 Jul 1986	TMP (10 off)	Sterile	
27 Aug 1986	TMP (63 off)	*P. mirabilis*	10^5
29 Oct 1986	TMP (63 on)	Sterile	
25 Nov 1986	TMP (90 on)	Sterile	
17 Dec 1986	TMP (22 off)	Sterile	
27 Jan 1987	TMP (63 off)	Sterile	
25 Mar 1987	TMP (119 off)	Sterile	
29 Apr 1987	TMP (154 off)	Sterile	
8 Jul 1987	TMP (224 off)	*P. mirabilis*	4×10^4

From Fowler, ref. 18.
TMP, trimethoprim

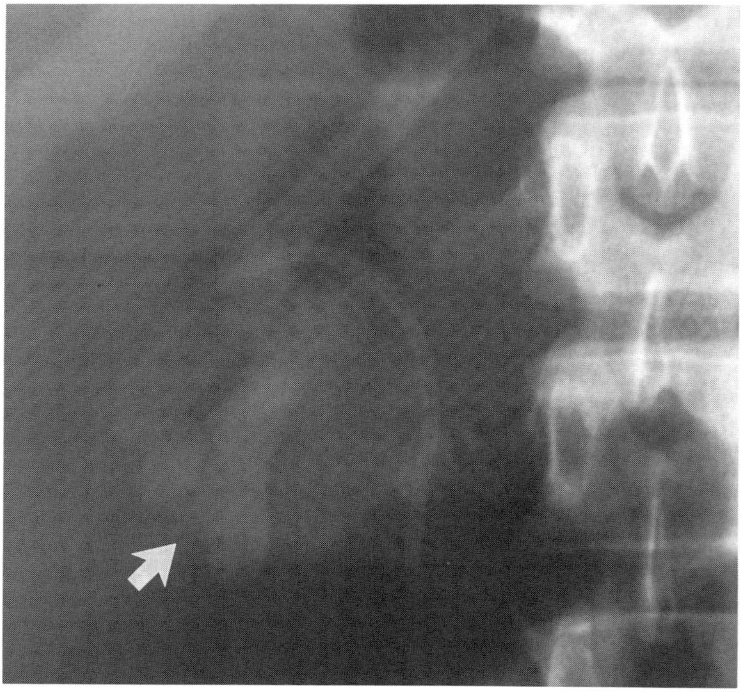

A

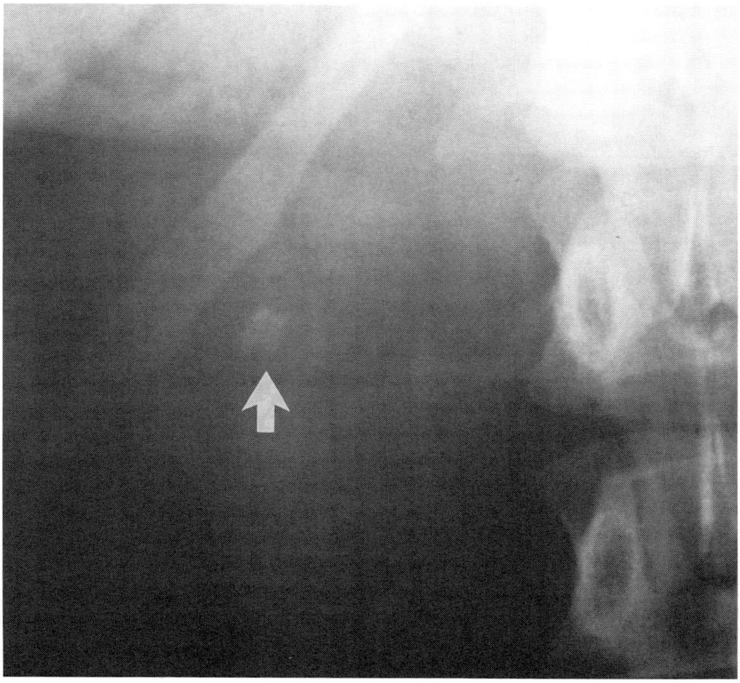

B

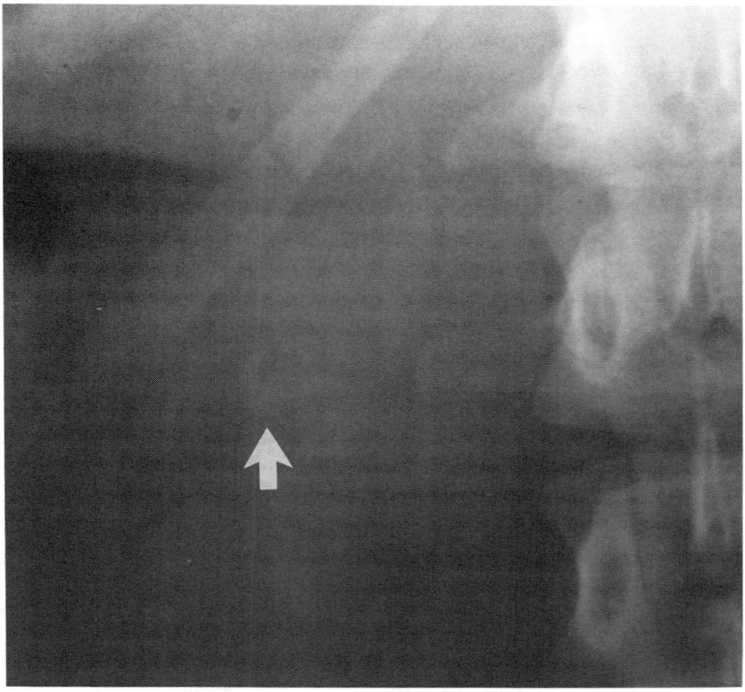

FIG. 6. Radiographs from case report 2. (**A**) Plain radiograph of abdomen showing branched right renal calculus (*arrow*) and ureteral stent. (**B**) Plain radiograph of abdomen showing residual renal stone fragments (*arrow*) 43 days after ESWL. (**C**) Plain radiograph of abdomen showing residual renal stone fragments (*arrow*) 12 months after ESWL. (From Fowler, ref. 18, with permission.)

of the stone was composed of struvite and approximately 40% was composed of carbonate apatite.

After 14 days of trimethoprim at full oral dosage, residual stone particles were still present in the collecting system. The drug was discontinued, and 35 days later a culture revealed *P. mirabilis* bacteriuria. The patient was then treated with a 3-month course of trimethoprim at full dosage. The urine was sterile during and 10 days after treatment, but *P. mirabilis* bacteriuria was again documented 2 months later. She then received another 3-month course of trimethoprim. After treatment the urine remained sterile for at least 154 days. However, *P. mirabilis* was isolated from a culture obtained 224 days after the most recent antimicrobial therapy. The appearance of the stone particles in the renal collecting system at this time is shown in Fig. 7b.

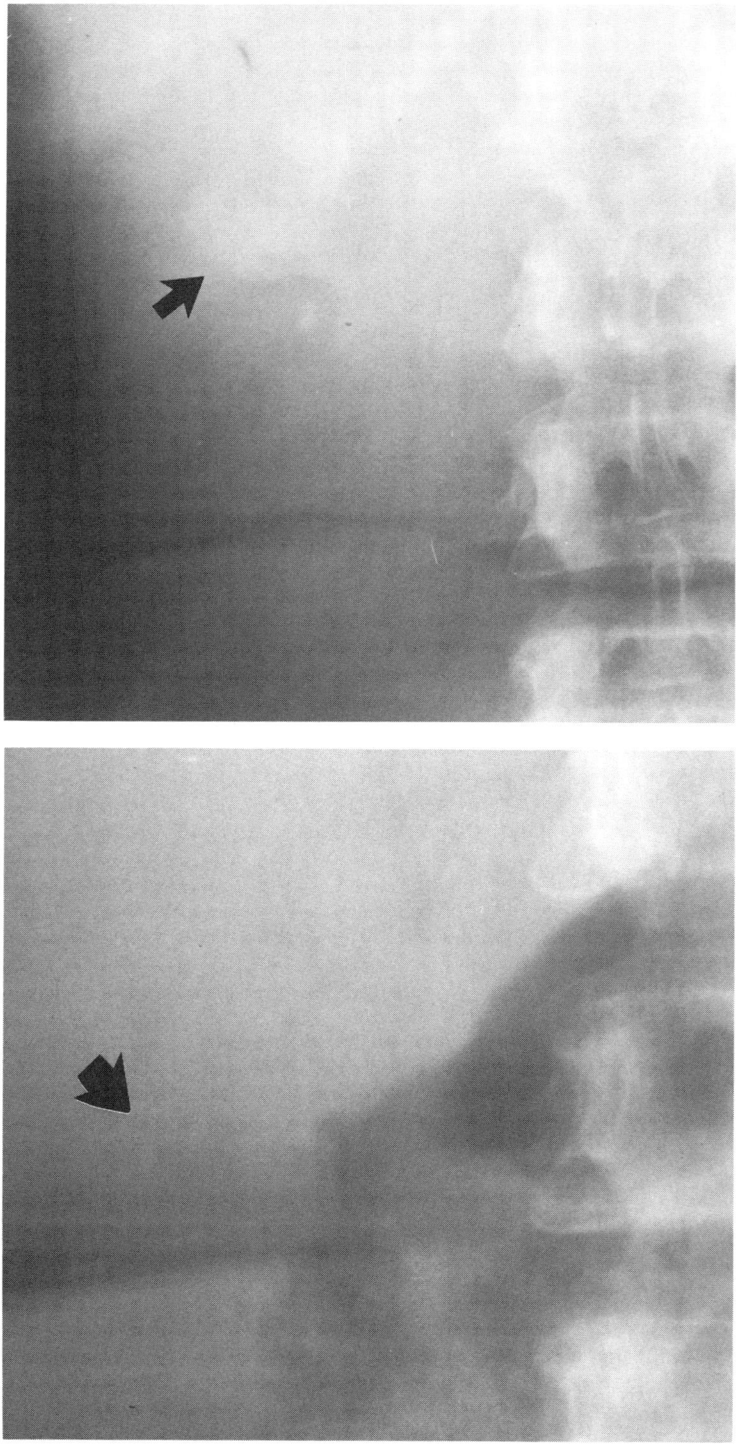

A

B

Comment

This is one of the three patients in our series of 22 women who were treated with ESWL monotherapy for infection stones and who had persistent bacteriuria following treatment. It is intriguing that the most recent *Proteus* infection occurred more than 6 months after stopping antimicrobial therapy. The biotype and antimicrobial susceptibilities of the *P. mirabilis* isolated from the four positive cultures were identical, and we have no reason to believe that these infections represented anything other than persistent bacteriuria. Prolonged bacteriologic surveillance following the treatment of infected renal calculi with ESWL, therefore, is clearly necessary.

The optimal management of a patient with residual stone particles and persistent bacteriuria after ESWL is not well established. Long-term suppressive antimicrobial therapy, hemiacidrin irrigations, or re-treatment with ESWL are reasonable therapeutic options.

REFERENCES

1. Blandy JP, Singh M. The case for a more aggressive approach to staghorn stones. *J Urol* 1976;115:505.
2. Sleight MW, Wickham JEA. Long-term follow-up of 100 cases of renal calculi. *Br J Urol* 1977;49:601.
3. Chute R, Suby HI. Prevalence and importance of urea-splitting bacterial infections of the urinary tract in the formation of calculi. *J Urol* 1940;44:590.
4. Fowler JE Jr. Bacteriology of branched renal calculi and accompanying urinary tract infection. *J Urol* 1984;131:213.
5. Nemoy NJ, Stamey TA. Surgical, bacteriological, and biochemical management of "infection stones." *JAMA* 1971;215:1470.
6. Griffith DP, Musher DM, Itin C. Urease. The primary cause of infection-induced urinary stones. *Invest Urol* 1976;13:346.
7. Rocha H, Santos LCS. Relapse of urinary tract infection in the presence of urinary tract calculi: the role of bacteria within the calculi. *J Med Microbiol* 1969;2:372.
8. Thompson RB, Stamey TA. Bacteriology of infected stones. *Urology* 1973;2:627.
9. Jones BD, Mobley HL. Genetic and biochemical diversity of ureases of Proteus, Providencia, and Morganella species isolated from urinary tract infection. *Infect Immun* 1987;55:2198.
10. Grenabo L, Claes G, Hedelin H, et al. Rapidly recurrent renal calculi caused by Ureaplasma urealyticum: a case report. *J Urol* 1986;135:995.
11. Pettersson S, Brorson JE, Grenabo L, et al. Ureaplasma urealyticum in infectious urinary tract stones. *Lancet* 1983;1:526.
12. Cardenas J, Quinn EL, Rooker G, et al. Single-dose cephalexin therapy for acute bacterial urinary tract infections and acute urethral syndrome with bladder bacteriuria. *Antimicrob Agents Chemother* 1986;29:383.

FIG. 7. Radiographs from case report 3. (**A**) Plain radiograph of the abdomen showing branched right renal calculus (*arrow*). (**B**) Plain radiograph of abdomen showing residual renal stone fragments (*arrow*) 18 months after ESWL. (From Fowler, ref. 18, with permission.)

13. Charlton CAC, Crowther A, Davies JG, et al. Three-day and ten-day chemotherapy for urinary tract infections in general practice. *Br Med J* 1976;1:124.
14. Iravani A, Pryor ND, Richard GA. Treatment of urinary tract infections with varying regimens of sulfisoxazole. *J Urol* 1983;130:484.
15. Jones RH. Single-dose and seven-day trimethoprim and co-trimoxazole in the treatment of urinary tract infection. *J Royal Coll Gen Prac* 1983;33:585.
16. Savard-Fenton M, Fenton BW, Reller LB, et al. Single-dose amoxicillin therapy with follow-up urine culture. *Am J Med* 1982;73:808.
17. Tolkoff-Rubin NE, Wilson ME, Zuromskis P, et al. Single-dose amoxicillin therapy of acute uncomplicated urinary tract infections in women. *Antimicrob Agents Chemother* 1984;25:626.
18. Fowler JE Jr. *Urinary tract infection and inflammation.* Chicago: Yearbook Medical Publishers; 1989:65.
19. Fowler JE Jr, Perkins T. Presentation, diagnosis and treatment of renal abscesses:1972–1988. *J Urol* 1994;151:847.
20. Michaels EK, Fowler JE Jr, Mariano M. Bacteriuria following extracorporeal shock wave lithotripsy of infection stones. *J Urol* 1988;140:254.
21. Rous SN, Turner WR. Retrospective study of 95 patients with staghorn calculus disease. *J Urol* 1977;118:902.
22. Patterson DE, Segura JW, LeRoy AJ. Long-term follow-up of patients treated by percutaneous ultrasonic lithotripsy for struvite staghorn calculi. *J Endourol* 1987;1:177.
23. Winfield HN, Clayman RV, Chaussy CG, Weyman PJ, Fuchs GJ, Lupu AN. Monotherapy of staghorn renal calculi: a comparative study between percutaneous nephrolithotomy and extracorporeal shock wave lithotripsy. *J Urol* 1988;139:895.
24. Newman DM, Scott JW, Lingeman JE. Two-year follow-up of patients treated with extracorporeal shock wave lithotripsy. *J Endourol* 1988;2:163.
25. Michaels EK, Fowler JE Jr. Extracorporeal shock wave lithotripsy for struvite renal calculi: prospective study with extended follow-up. *J Urol* 1991;146:728.
26. Nemoy NJ, Stamey TA. Use of hemiacidrin in management of infection stones. *J Urol* 1976;116:693.
27. Dretler SP, Pfister RC. Primary dissolution therapy of struvite calculi. *J Urol* 1984;131:861.
28. Blaivas JG, Pais VM, Spellman RM. Chemolysis of residual stone fragments after extensive surgery for staghorn calculi. *Urology* 1975;6:681.
29. Fam B, Rossier AB, Yalla S, et al. The role of hemiacidrin in the management of renal stones in spinal cord injury patients. *J Urol* 1976;116:696.
30. Jacobs SC, Gittes RF. Dissolution of residual renal calculi with hemiacidrin. *J Urol* 1976;115:2.
31. Klein RS, Cattolica EV, Rankin KN. Hemiacidrin renal irrigation: complications and successful management. *J Urol* 1982;128:241.
32. Royle G, Smith JC. Recurrence of infected calculi following postoperative renal irrigation with stone solvent. *Br J Urol* 1976;48:531.
33. Silverman DE, Stamey TA. Management of infection stones: the Stanford experience. *Medicine* 1983;62:44.
34. Hovelius B, Mardh PA. On the diagnosis of coagulase-negative staphylococci with emphasis on Staphylococcus saprophyticus. *Acta Pathol Microbiol Scand* 1977;85B:427.
35. Olafsen LD, Melby K. Urinary tract infection with septicaemia due to Staphylococcus saprophyticus in a patient with a ureteric calculus. *J Infect* 1986;13:92.
36. Fowler JE Jr. Staphylococcus saprophyticus as the cause of infected urinary calculus. *Ann Intern Med* 1985;102:342.

Antibiotic Therapy in Urology,
edited by S. Grant Mulholland, M.D.,
Lippincott-Raven Publishers, Philadelphia © 1996.

Chapter 12

Bacteriuria in Spinal Cord Injured Patients

*Gregor Reid, †Heather J. L. Brooks,
‡Hanna Bialkowska-Hobrzanska, and §Miguel Valvano

**‡§ The University of Western Ontario, London, Ontario, Canada N6A 4U2;
†Department of Microbiology, Otago University, Dunedin, New Zealand*

INTRODUCTION

Urinary tract infections (UTI) constitute a sizable problem, causing morbidity and sometimes mortality, in patients requiring acute and long-term care and those with spinal cord injury (1–6). In general, the acute and long-term treatment of UTI in spinal cord-injured (SCI) patients has been similar to the treatment of otherwise healthy women, in that the same antimicrobial agents and dosages are used. However, recent research indicates that the pathogenesis of UTI in SCI patients is different from that in otherwise healthy women, and that its management should be evaluated carefully.

PATHOGENESIS

The pathogenesis of UTI in adult women has been covered elsewhere in this text, but in summary, there is some evidence to indicate that bacteria use various mechanisms to adhere to the bladder mucosa and also multiply in urine, thereby causing disease (7,8). The use of antibiotics and the induction of an effective host response, in combination with micturition, leads to clearance of the organisms and "cure" of the patient. However, in SCI patients the infection process appears to involve heavy colonization of the bladder mucosa in a biofilm mode (dense layers of bacteria surrounded by glycocalyx material). This makes traditional diagnosis more difficult, as conventional techniques utilize urine, where planktonic (free-floating), not adherent, organisms reside. Often, urine culture can be negative, when in fact the organisms are colonizing surfaces (9,10).

While the use of intermittent catheterization can reduce the infection rate (11), the biofilms that form on the mucosa are not eradicated by conventional therapy (9), and the evidence to support this conclusion from 23 patients and 69 specimens is quite convincing (9,12,13).

The possibility that the organisms infecting SCI patients have different pathogenic properties from those infecting otherwise healthy adult women has not been investigated, but it appears unlikely. A study of uropathogens from elderly women showed that the organisms had similar properties as those infecting young women, implying that it was the status of the host that conferred different responses to the bacteria (14).

Many SCI patients become infected in the hospital, and although catheter-associated bacteriuria is often polymicrobial (15), in our experience with patients using intermittent catheterization, *Escherichia coli* causes the majority of the infections (9). The diverse expression of adhesins in these organisms, including type 1, 1C, P, S, and G fimbriae, and M, Dr, and X adhesins, has been shown to affect host-parasite interactions (16–23). In addition, the expression of certain O serogroups, 2, 4, 6, 8, 18ab, and 75, high K-antigen titer, and production of hemolysin are important contributors to pathogenesis (24,25).

Our recent experience has shown that *Enterococcus faecalis* is a particularly pathogenic organism in the urinary tract of SCI patients (26), and similar findings have been reported by others (27, 28). There is some evidence to indicate that carbohydrate adhesins play a role in enterococcal colonization and infection (29). Molecular typing has verified that certain clones can disseminate among many patients in one unit over a period of 18 months (Bialkowska-Hobrzanska and Reid, manuscript in preparation). The problem can be further amplified if the enterococci are resistant to vancomycin, aminoglycosides, penicillins, and many other antimicrobial agents (30,31). These organisms cause potentially fatal blood and cerebral spinal infections (32), and in some cases they are resistant to all available antimicrobials (33). In vitro studies have shown that vancomycin, erythromycin, chloramphenicol, gentamicin, and streptomycin resistance can be transferred from *E. faecalis* to *Staphylococcus aureus* (34). As staphylococci are prevalent in the urogenital tract, this poses a serious threat to infection control. Another molecular and epidemiologic study of multiresistant *Serratia marcescens* has shown that pathogens can be a reservoir for infection, including UTI, in SCI units (35). Preliminary results obtained in London, Canada, on nine enterococcal strains isolated from SCI patients have shown that antibiotic resistance in planktonic form is prevalent, including resistance against norfloxacin, ampicillin, gentamicin, tetracycline, penicillin, and streptomycin (Table 1). Polymerase chain reaction (PCR) was used to detect VanA, VanB, and VanC phenotypes, but so far no isolate from Parkwood Hospital in London, Ontario, has developed resistance to vancomycin.

Table 1. *Antibiotic resistance among nine enterococcal strains isolated from spinal cord injury patients with bacteriuria*

Isolate	Fm	Nor	Tet	Pen	Amp	Gm	Sm	Van1[a]	Van2[b]
04	S	R	R	S	S	S	R	S	S
05	S	S	R	S	S	S	R	S	S
06	S	S	R	S	S	R	R	S	S
09	S	R	R	S	S	S	R	S	S
10	S	S	R	S	S	R	R	S	S
12[c]	S	R	S	R	R	S	R	S	S
12	S	R	S	R	R	S	R	S	S
16	S	S	R	S	S	R	R	S	S
19	S	R	R	S	S	S	R	S	S
23	S	S	R	S	S	R	R	S	S
Laboratory Proficiency Testing Program (LPTP) Control for vancomycin resistance									R

Fm, nitrofurantoin; Nor, norfloxacin; Tet, tetracycline; Pen, penicillin G; Amp, ampicillin; Gm, gentamicin; Sm, streptomycin; Van, vancomycin; S, susceptible; R, resistant.

[a]Vitek test.

[b]Agar dilution test.

[c]Two colonies of isolate 12 were examined.

However, moderate susceptibility to vancomycin has been found, raising the concern that resistant strains may soon emerge.

Vancomycin is a glycopeptide that inhibits bacterial mucopeptide biosynthesis. The mechanisms of resistance appear to involve structural genes VanA, VanH, and VanC as well as plasmid-encoded genes and a putative protein VanR (36,37). A recent study has shown that exposure to vancomycin can induce surface changes in gram-positive cocci and rods as well as gram-negative rods, potentially preventing entry of antimicrobial agents into the cell (38). This coincides with the finding that the presence of glycine substantially lowered the vancomycin minimal inhibitory concentrations (MICs), implying that amino acids, presumably on the surface of the bacteria, interfere with the mechanism(s) of acquired vancomycin resistance in enterococci (39). Another study of gram-positive organisms (lactobacilli) showed that resistance to vancomycin correlated with the presence of hydrophilic components on the cell surface (40). Further studies combining surface, molecular, and adhesion properties and antibiograms are required to understand more fully the extent of the problem that enterococci pose to the urinary tract of SCI patients.

SIGNS AND SYMPTOMS

The cause(s) of signs and symptoms in UTI patients are not well known at present. In SCI patients, it is particularly difficult to use signs and symptoms to assess the status of bacteriuria. Factors such as spasticity, foul-smelling urine, fatigue, and fever can be of assistance in diagnosis of infection. Often, the presence of these factors in combination with significant bacteriuria (>10^5 organisms per milliliter of urine) leads to treatment of infection, whereas a patient who lacks signs and symptoms goes untreated, as will be discussed later.

It would seem likely that characteristics of the bacteria, including their by-products, are important in the induction of signs and symptoms of infection. Host factors are also likely to be part of the process. For example, it has been shown that interleukin-6 and antibodies are produced in response to bacterial invasion of the urinary tract (41–43). There is some evidence to suggest that the lipopolysaccharides (LPS) of Enterobacteriaceae also stimulate a host response and may induce signs and symptoms of UTI (44). In addition, antibiotic exposure often causes increased release of LPS endotoxin, but the implications for the patient in respect to bladder damage remain to be examined.

Preliminary evidence from our latest in vitro and in vivo studies suggests that it is possible that toxicity could be related to signs and symptoms of UTI and that the numbers of adherent bacteria per cell might be important. Physicians have often stated that it would be a major breakthrough if they were able to predict at what time a given patient will develop symptomatic infection. By doing so, it might be possible to better manage antibiotic therapy. In an effort to address this issue, specimens were collected from SCI patients. It was discovered that in 63% of asymptomatic episodes, the bacterial adhesion counts were < 20 per bladder cell, whereas in 81% of cases with at least one sign and one symptom of UTI, adhesion counts were > 20 per cell. This has led us to propose that a cut-off at 20 bacteria per cell may suggest to a physician that the patient is at this time more likely to develop clinical UTI (26). Further studies will be needed to determine whether this cut-off point is the most appropriate in the majority of cases.

TREATMENT

When bacteria are detected in the bladder, the patient is not necessarily given antibiotics. A consensus report from the National Institute on Disability and Rehabilitation Research (NIDRR) (45) recommended that symptomatic UTI should be treated with antibiotics for 7 to 14 days, and that asymptomatic bacteriuria (ABU) need not be treated with antibiotics. It is not clear what scientific basis exists for these conclusions. In addition, this consensus was published prior to the discovery and report of the presence of bacterial biofilms on the bladder cells of SCI patients.

Presumably, the clinical reasons for not treating ABU are the concern over the emergence of drug-resistant organisms and a realization that reinfection or recolonization is probably inevitable and may occur with onset of symptoms, and that no organ deterioration will occur (46). It was also stated in the NIDRR report that the treatment of UTI could be commenced without waiting for culture results, apparently because the identification of the infecting species does not alter the selection or dosage of the drug. Several studies leave these NIDRR conclusions open to questioning. The NIDRR consensus is incorrect in assuming that any antibiotic can be used. Firstly, no antibiotic appears to resolve the situation, if one evaluates the follow-up urine cultures (47) and pathogens adherent to bladder cells (9). Secondly, agents such as co-trimoxazole, the most commonly prescribed antimicrobial for UTI in our experience, would not be effective against a large number of uropathogens, especially enterococci, which are common uropathogens in many hospital settings (13,48). The consensus report is correct in the sense that treatment need not wait for a laboratory report. However, the reason is different from that expressed in the report: the MIC data for a drug against a microbe are of no real value for the eradication of bacterial biofilms (9,10,49). To correct this flaw, microbiology laboratories would have to test for the biofilm elimination concentrations (BEC), but this technology is not available commercially.

When active therapy is administered to treat UTI, it can be useful in eradicating some, but perhaps not all, bacteria from the bladder. However, antibiotic therapy does not change a patient's susceptibility to reinfection; that is, on cessation of treatment, the bladder cells are still available to bacteria for colonization (50). Until recently, no antibiotic tested has been shown to penetrate bacterial biofilms on surfaces in vitro or in vivo (10,51,52). Our in vivo studies confirmed the lack of effect of various antibiotics on adherent biofilms in SCI patients. The only change that was found with treatment was the loss of symptoms in 52% of cases. The antibiotics appeared to have removed the planktonic organisms, and presumably these were, at least in part, responsible for the signs and symptoms of infection (13). This may be a result of a reduction in total bacterial load, but to date almost no information is available on what actually causes symptoms such as frequency, urgency, and dysuria. It would seem logical to investigate these factors, and to understand the mechanisms with a view to developing interference therapy.

It is clear that current approaches to antibiotic prophylaxis and therapy, often based on reports in the 1970s (53), are not fully effective when dense adherent organisms are present in biofilms (12). The possibility that fluoroquinolones could be used to clear these organisms is worthy of investigation. If the intent is to eradicate bacteria from the bladder, then an appropriate antibiotic should be used. The effectiveness of fluoroquinolones has been supported by studies showing that these agents are able to kill a significant portion of adherent bacteria (26). Ciprofloxacin is especially effective at reducing the number of adherent organisms on patients' cells to < 20 per cell, deemed to be a level less serious for the prognosis. Another in vitro investigation has shown that ciprofloxacin is particularly effective at preventing adhesion and eradicating *Pseudomonas aeruginosa* adherent to urinary catheters (54). In a study of multiple sclerosis patients with neurogenic bladders who required transurethral maneuvers, it was found that ciprofloxacin (100- and 500-mg oral doses twice daily for 4 days) provides excellent coverage without inducing bacterial resistance to any high level (55).

The effectiveness of another oral fluoroquinolone, norfloxacin, has been demonstrated in outpatients with neurogenic bladder secondary to SCI (56). While the use of 14-day therapy appears excessive and only planktonic organisms were examined, that study did suggest that norfloxacin is a reasonable choice of agent.

The use of antibiotics for longer than 3 days should also be reconsidered in relation to UTI. It is not unusual for antibiotics, especially the fluoroquinolones, to eradicate planktonic bacteria from the bladder in 1 to 3 days (57,58). Seven-day therapy with some agents disrupts the normal urogenital flora and may increase the risk of reinfection and emergence of drug-resistant organisms (59). The treatment of infection for 14 days appears to be an overuse of antibiotics, especially now that we recognize that the agents do not eradicate the biofilm bacteria and some increase the patient's susceptibility to reinfection (59,60).

Concerns arise if uropathogens develop resistance, particularly against fluoroquinolones. This issue was raised by Waites et al. (61), although the article was written in such a way that it was difficult to understand fully what was happening. The suggestion was that there were high levels of resistance to ciprofloxacin, yet the effectiveness of the assay was not stated, no data were given for norfloxacin, and no correlation was presented between so-called resistance and clinical outcome for the patient. One would also ask why an antibiotic was prescribed if the organism was resistant. Nevertheless, a useful point was made that asymptomatic bacteriuria ($>10^5$ colonies per milliliter, >10 urinary leukocytes per high-power field) was difficult to eradicate with 7 to 14 days of therapy using norfloxacin, co-trimoxazole, ciprofloxacin, ampicillin, cephalothin, and other agents (as low as 54% sterility midtreatment), and relapses or reinfection occurred by day 16 following therapy. The report made no mention of bacterial biofilms, but it seems likely that these were present in some, if not all, of the patients. Clearly, an evaluation of antibiotic usage is worthy of close scrutiny, as well as agents used that can eradicate bacteria from the bladder cells and urine.

THE OUTCOME OF BACTERIAL PERSISTENCE IN THE BLADDER

If, as has been recommended by NIDRR, ABU is not to be treated, what is the outcome for the patient? A state-of-the-art review has rightly pointed out that the mere presence of bacteriuria in the urinary tract is abnormal and does predispose SCI and non-SCI persons to increased morbidity and mortality (62). The authors argue that the treatment of UTI can be justified to impact on symptoms and prevent further complications, but that the development of drug resistance and the cost prohibit treatment in ABU. In our study of SCI patients, we showed that biofilm formation associated with UTI and ABU caused a significant drop in bladder cell viability and a large increase in leukocyte response (26). The fact that there

Table 2. *Summary of bladder cell viability results*

				Change in % cell viability[c]	
Organism	Fluid[a]	Time, h	Adhesion[b]	Add cells[d]	Add supernatant[e]
E. faecalis[f]	Broth	1	18	-15.6	-5.6
		2	51	-21.6	-5.4
		4	69	-25.4	-8.7
	Urine	1	-[g]	-15.2	-11.6
		2	-	-18.9	-12.6
		4	-	-19.5	-11.2
E. coli[f]	Broth	1	43	-3.9	-5.0
		2	63	-5.7	-5.4
		4	114	-9.9	-7.5
	Urine	1	29	-10.3	-8.6
		2	50	-13.8	-9.0
		4	93	-9.3	-7.4
Lactobacillus	Broth	1	8	0	0
		2	26	-6.7	0
		4	37	-3.4	0
	Urine	1	13	-8.6	-1.0
		2	28	-18.0	-8.8
		4	44	-15.2	-10.9

[a]The suspending solution in which the experiments were carried out.
[b]The mean number of bacteria that adhered to 50 bladder cells after in vitro incubation with the organisms.
[c]Mean change in % cell viability compared with 3 *E. faecalis*, 5 *E. coli*, and 5 *Lactobacillus* sp (acting as controls as they are not regularly regarded as pathogenic to the bladder) after 1, 2, and 4 h incubation of whole cells and growth supernatants with uroepithelial cells harvested from healthy premenopausal women.
[d]Change in epithelial cell viability when whole bacterial cells were added to suspensions of bladder epithelial cells.
[e]Change in epithelial cell viability when supernatants from bacterial cultures were added to suspensions of bladder epithelial cells.
[f]The killing effect of *E. coli* and *E. faecalis* pathogens was 83% overall greater than that of *Lactobacillus*, indicating that the latter had much less effect on cell viability. Interestingly, *E. faecalis* appeared to have a more detrimental effect on bladder cells than *E. coli*.
[g]Results not available.

was increased cell death illustrates, at least in part, the damage that these organisms confer on the host. Further in vitro studies have provided some evidence to suggest that *E. coli* and *E. faecalis* can produce substances that adversely affect bladder cell viability (Table 2). At present, we are investigating the possible role of bacterial components, such as lipopolysaccharides, in killing bladder epithelial cells.

It is still not yet clear to what extent the level of bacterial colonization affects the cell killing, nor which factors are responsible. In addition, more extensive studies are required to verify which uropathogens are particularly toxic to cell viability, and to compare cells from SCI patients and controls. It should be noted that the adhesion to uroepithelial cells of *E. coli* and *E. faecalis* can be very high, even within a few hours.

Another study has shown that the adhesion of *E. coli* to cells facilitates the presentation of bacterial components that cause inflammation in the tissues (63). Although pyuria does not prove that invasion has occurred (5), its gross presence places the patient at risk of increased morbidity (64,65). By not treating the patient, the physician is caught in a difficult dilemma. Clearly, as Stover et al. (62) suggested, newer methods of treatment and management are required to solve this situation.

ECONOMICS OF TREATMENT

One of the considerations when using fluoroquinolones is their higher cost compared with co-trimoxazole, which is often used to prevent and treat UTI. However, in our experience the use of the latter does not eradicate biofilms; and prophylaxis with this agent appears to correlate with more virulent organisms subsequently infecting the hosts (26). A study of 302 patients using clean intermittent catheterization has shown that those using anti-infectives had fewer episodes of bacteriuria but significantly more clinical UTI; (66). A very important study of 129 SCI patients has shown that once-daily co-trimoxazole does reduce the incidence of UTI, but numerous breakthrough infections occurred, many adverse events took place, and high numbers of drug-resistant organisms were found in the bladder, urethra, and rectum (67).

In order to control the cost of therapy for UTI, it has been recommended that oral rather than parenteral antibiotics should be used (68). It was also pointed out that overall cost savings can be achieved if the most effective agents against bacteriuria are used, regardless of their cost. We believe that our findings on bacterial biofilms and the ability of fluoroquinolones to penetrate them provide a scientific basis for making cost-effective recommendations regarding which antibiotics should be preferred.

A recent retrospective health economics study of 81 SCI patients who were admitted to one hospital wing was undertaken to determine whether the use of prophylactic antibiotics caused a reduction in the incidence of symptomatic and asymptomatic infection, affected time to discharge, improved well-being, and influenced hospitalization costs. In addition, the study examined the cost of acquiring, preparing, administering, and monitoring the agents as well as failure rates and side effects. Preliminary analysis suggests that time to first infection is not changed when patients are given prophylaxis, and "cure" may be faster with fluoroquinolones (manuscript in preparation). If a study indeed shows that effective treatment of UTI can be achieved with certain antibiotics, and that the costs of treating infection are similar to those incurred using prophylaxis, it might be argued that using drugs such as fluoroquinolones, and stopping co-trimoxazole prophylaxis, would not raise expenditure. That being the case, a review of drug use in SCI patients could be warranted. The economic impact can be very significant, as shown by a multicenter study of 766 patients, in which the switching to oral ciprofloxacin from parenteral antibiotics resulted in an estimated cost saving of $980,246, attributable mainly to shorter hospital stay and reduced dosage (69).

PARALLELS WITH NEUROGENIC DISORDERS

There is a case to be made that UTI in SCI patients has some similarities to infections in patients with neurogenic bladder disease and infections in the total patient population with residual urine volumes. The bladder of a spinal cord-injured patient can be viewed as a model in which voiding is abnormal and urine is a constant nutritional source for organisms that ascend into the bladder. From the perspective of an organism, this is an ideal habitat for colonization, survival, and growth. Not only are urinary and mucous nutrients available, but host surfaces, material surfaces (in the case of indwelling catheters), and damaged tissues (from trauma upon catheterization) act as sites for establishment. Thus, it should not be surprising to find the organisms living in a quite different mode from those that multiply and attempt to disseminate primarily as planktonic organisms in healthy adult bladders. There, they compete with the full voiding process, active host-immune responses, possibly larger fluid intake, and antibiotics with proven efficacy against free-floating bacteria. The dilemma is that for SCI patients, even if the therapy can eradicate biofilm organisms, colonization simply returns on cessation of treatment.

THE FUTURE

In the future, we must concentrate efforts on more fully understanding the basic mechanisms of host-bacterial interactions in SCI and neurogenic bladder patients before devising management techniques. At present, long-term therapy with antibiotics such as nitrofurantoin or co-trimoxazole is claimed to be our only weapon (70). The potential to insert "nonpathogens" into the bladder has been explored previously (71–73) and is being studied further. The rationale is that bacterial colonization is inevitable, so why not establish organisms that will not damage the host?

Clearly, concerns over infection must be weighed against the need for surgical interventions and the ultimate goal of preservation of renal function (62). In the future, the urologist will be asked to become more and more knowledgeable about pathogenic bacteria and their virulence properties, indigenous flora and their protective properties, and how and when antimicrobial therapy should be applied.

ACKNOWLEDGMENTS

This chapter was prepared with the support of a grant from the Natural Sciences and Engineering Research Council, Medical Research Council, and in part from Bayer Canada. The resources provided by the Department of Microbiology at the University of Otago are appreciated. The technical assistance of Ms. Wei Zhong, Ms. Lydia Dafoe, and Ms. Dominique Lam is acknowledged.

REFERENCES

1. Warren JW, Tenney JH, Hoopes JM, Muncie HL, Anthony WC. A prospective microbiological study of bacteriuria in patients with chronic indwelling urethral catheters. *J Infect Dis* 1982;146:719–723.
2. Warren JW, Damron D, Tenney JH, Hoopes JM, Deforge B, Muncie HL Jr. Fever, bacteremia and death as complications of bacteriuria in women with long-term urethral catheters. *J Infect Dis* 1987;155:1151–1158.
3. Stickler DJ, Chawla JC. An appraisal of antibiotic policies for urinary tract infections in patients with spinal cord injuries undergoing long-term intermittent catheterization. *Paraplegia* 1988;26:215–225.
4. Johnson JR, Stamm WE. Urinary tract infections in women: diagnosis and treatment. *Ann Intern Med* 1989;111:906–917.
5. Gribble MJ, Puterman ML, McCallum NM. Pyuria: its relationship to bacteriuria in spinal cord injured patients on intermittent catheterization. *Arch Phys Med Rehabil* 1989;70:376–379.
6. Montgomerie JZ, Chan E, Gilmore DS, Canawati HN, Sapico FL. Low mortality among patients with spinal cord injury and bacteremia. *Rev Infect Dis* 1991;13:867–871.
7. Reid G, Brooks HJL. The use of double staining techniques for investigating bacterial attachment to mucopolysaccharide-coated epithelial cells. *Stain Technol* 1982;57:5–11.
8. Reid G, Sobel JD. Bacterial adherence in the pathogenesis of urinary tract infection: a review. *Rev Infect Dis* 1987;9:470–487.
9. Reid G, Charbonneau-Smith R, Lam D, Lacerte M, Kang YS, Hayes KC. Bacterial biofilm formation in the urinary bladder of spinal cord injured patients. *Paraplegia* 1992;30:711–717.
10. Reid G, Denstedt JD, Kang YS, Lam D, Naus C. Bacterial adhesion and biofilm formation on ureteral stents in vitro and in vivo. *J Urol* 1992;148:1592–1594.

11. Kuhn W, Rist M, Zaech GA. Intermittent urethral self-catheterization: long term results (bacteriologic evolution, continence, acceptance, complications). *Paraplegia* 1991;29:222–232.
12. Reid G. Do antibiotics clear bladder infections? *J Urol* 1994;152:865–867.
13. Reid G, Kang YS, Lacerte M, Tieszer C, Hayes KC. Bacterial biofilm formation on the bladder epithelium of spinal cord injured patients. II. Toxic outcome on cell viability. *Paraplegia* 1993;31:494–499.
14. Reid G, Zorzitto ML, Bruce AW, Jewett MAS, Chan RCY, Costerton JW. The pathogenesis of urinary tract infection in the elderly: the role of bacterial adherence to uroepithelial cells. *Curr Microbiol* 1984;11:67–72.
15. Rahav G, Pinco E, Silbaq F, Bercovier H. Molecular epidemiology of catheter-associated bacteriuria in nursing home patients. *J Clin Microbiol* 1994;32:1031–1034.
16. Hacker J, Schmidt G, Hughes C, Knapp S, Marget M, Goebel W. Cloning and characterization of genes involved in production of mannose-resistant, neuraminidase-susceptible (X) fimbriae from a uropathogenic 06:K15:H31 Escherichia coli strain. *Infect Immun* 1985;47:434–440.
17. Hagberg L, Jodal U, Korhonen TK, Lidin-Janson G, Lindberg U, Svanborg Eden C. Adhesion, hemagglutination and virulence of Escherichia coli causing urinary tract infections. *Infect Immun* 1981;31:564–570.
18. Hultgren SJ, Porter TN, Schaeffer AJ, Duncan JL. Role of type 1 pili and effects of phase variation on lower urinary tract infections produced by Escherichia coli. *Infect Immun* 1985;50:370–377.
19. Kallenius G, Mollby R, Winberg J. Adhesion of Escherichia coli to periurethral cells correlated to mannose-resistant agglutination of human erythrocytes. *FEMS Microbiol Lett* 1979;5:295–299.
20. Kist ML, Salit IE, Hofmann T. Purification and characterization of the Dr hemagglutinins expressed by two uropathogenic Escherichia coli strains. *Infect Immun* 1990;58:695–702.
21. Rhen M, Klemm P, Korhonen TK. Identification of two new hemagglutinins of Escherichia coli, N-acetyl-D-glucosamine-specific fimbriae and a blood group M-specific agglutinin, by cloning the corresponding genes in Escherichia coli K-12. *J Bacteriol* 1986;168:1234–1242.
22. Vaisanen V, Korhonen TK, Jokinen M, Gahmberg CG, Ehnholm C. Blood group M specific haemagglutinin in pyelonephritogenic Escherichia coli. *Lancet* 1982;1:1192.
23. Vaisanen-Rhen V, Korhonen TK, Finne J. Novel cell-binding activity specific for N-acetyl-D-glucosamine in an Escherichia coli strain. *FEBS Lett* 1983;159:223–236.
24. Brooks HJL, O'Grady F, McSherry MA, Cattell WR. Uropathogenic properties of Escherichia coli in recurrent urinary-tract infection. *J Med Microbiol* 1980;13:57–68.
25. Kaijser B. Immunology of Escherichia coli: K antigen and its relation to urinary-tract infection. *J Infect Dis* 1973;127:670–677.
26. Reid G, Dafoe L, Valvano M, Lacerte M, Delaney G, Hayes KC. Ability of fluoroquinolones to penetrate bacterial biofilms on bladder cells of spinal cord injured patients. *Paraplegia* 1994;32:468–472.
27. Felmingham D, Wilson APR, Quintana AI, Gruneberg RN. Enterococcus species in urinary tract infection. *Clin Infect Dis* 1992;15:295–301.
28. Murray BE. The life and times of the enterococcus. *Clin Microbiol Rev* 1990;3:46–65.
29. Jett BD, Huycke MM, Gilmore MS. Virulence of enterococci. *Clin Microbiol Rev* 1994;7:462–478.
30. Murray BE. New aspects of antimicrobial resistance and the resulting therapeutic dilemmas. *J Infect Dis* 1991;163:1184–1194.
31. Willey BM, Kreiswirth BN, Simor AE, Williams G, Scriver SR, Phillips A, Low DE. Detection of vancomycin resistance in Enterococcus species. *J Clin Microbiol* 1992;30:1621–1624.
32. Haglund LA, Flournoy DJ, Gilmore MS, Huycke MM. Enterococcus: an old pathogen with new tricks. *J Okla State Med Assoc* 1991;84:305–309.
33. Frieden TR, Munsiff SS, Low DE, Willey BM, Williams G, Faur Y, Eisner W, Warren S, Kreiswirth B. Emergence of vancomycin-resistant enterococci in New York City. *Lancet* 1993;342:76–79.
34. Noble WC, Virani Z, Cree RG. Co-transfer of vancomycin and other resistance genes from Enterococcus faecalis NCTC 12201 to Staphylococcus aureus. *FEMS Microbiol Lett* 1992;72:195–198.

35. Simor AE, Ramage L, Wilcox L, Bull SB, Bialkowska-Hobrzanska H. Molecular and epidemiologic study of multi-resistant Serratia marcescens infections in a spinal cord injury rehabilitation unit. *Infect Control Hosp Epidemiol* 1988;9:20–27.
36. Handwerger S, Discotto L, Thanassi J, Pucci MJ. Insertional inactivation of a gene which controls expression of vancomycin resistance on plasmid pHKK100. *FEMS Microbiol Lett* 1992;71:11–14.
37. Leclercq R, Dutka-Malen S, Duval J, Courvalin P. Vancomycin resistance gene vanC is specific to Enterococcus gallinarum. *Antimicrob Agents Chemother* 1992;36:2005–2008.
38. Cuperus PL, van der Mei HC, Reid G, Bruce AW, Khoury AE, van der Kuijl-Booij M, Busscher HJ. Effects of ciprofloxacin and vancomycin on physico-chemical surface properties of S. epidermidis, E. coli and L. casei and L. acidophilus. *Microbios* 1995;82:49–67.
39. Zarlenga LJ, Gilmore MS, Sahm DF. Effects of amino acids on expression of enterococcal vancomycin resistance. *Antimicrob Agents Chemother* 1992;36:902–905.
40. Tomeczek T, Reid G, Cuperus PL, McGroarty JA, van der Mei HC, Bruce AW, Khoury AH, Busscher HJ. Correlation between hydrophobicity and resistance to nonoxynol-9 and vancomycin for urogenital isolates of lactobacilli. *FEMS Microbiol Lett* 1992;94:101–104.
41. Montgomerie JZ, Guerra DA, Schick DG, Gilmore DS, Tabatabai MF, Morrow JW. Pseudomonas urinary tract infection in patients with spinal cord injury. *J Am Paraplegia Soc* 1989;12:8–10.
42. Galloway A, Green HT, Menon KK, Gardner BP, Pemberton S, Krishnan KR. Antibody coated bacteria in urine of patients with recent spinal injury. *J Clin Pathol* 1990;43:953–956.
43. Hedges S, Anderson P, Lidin-Janson G, de Man P, Svanborg C. Interleukin-6 response to deliberate colonization of the human urinary tract with gram-negative bacteria. *Infect Immun* 1991;59:421–427.
44. Hurley JC, Louis WJ, Tosolini FA, Carlin JB. Antibiotic-induced release of endotoxin in chronically bacteriuric patients. *Antimicrob Agents Chemother* 1991;35:2388–2394.
45. National Institute on Disability and Rehabilitation Research Consensus Statement. The prevention and management of urinary tract infections among people with spinal cord injuries. *J Am Paraplegia Soc* 1992;15:194–204.
46. Sotolongo JR Jr, Koleiiat N. Significance of asymptomatic bacteriuria in spinal cord injury patients on condom catheter. *J Urol* 1990;143:979–980.
47. Montgomerie JZ, Gilmore DB, Canawati HN, Morrow JW. Ceftazidime in treatment of urinary tract infection in patients with spinal cord injury: comparison with moxalactam. *Urology* 1990;35:93–95.
48. Preston C, Bruce AW, Reid G. Antibiotic resistance of urinary pathogens isolated from patients attending the Toronto Hospital between 1986 and 1990. *J Hosp Infect* 1992;22:129–135.
49. Reid G, Khoury A, Neumann AW, Bruce AW. Components involved in biomaterial-related infections. *AUA Update Series* 1992;18:138–144.
50. Reid G, Bruce AW, Beheshti M. Effect of antibiotic treatment on receptivity of uroepithelial cells to uropathogens. *Can J Microbiol* 1988;34:327–331
51. Nickel JC, Wright JB, Ruseka I, Marrie TJ, Whitfield C, Costerton JW. Antibiotic resistance of Pseudomonas aeruginosa colonizing a urinary catheter in vitro. *Eur J Clin Microbiol* 1985;4:213–218.
52. Costerton JW, Cheng K-J, Geesey GG, Ladd TI, Nickel JC, Dasgupta M, Marrie TJ. Bacterial biofilms in nature and disease. *Annu Rev Microbiol* 1987;41:435–464.
53. Stamey TA, Condy M, Mihara G. Prophylactic efficacy of nitrofurantoin macrocrystals and trimethoprim-sulfamethoxazole in urinary infections. *N Engl J Med* 1977;96:78–84.
54. Reid G, Sharma S, Advikolanu K, Martin RA, Bruce AW. Effect of ciprofloxacin, norfloxacin and ofloxacin in vitro on the adhesion and survival of Pseudomonas aeruginosa on urinary catheters. *Antimicrob Agents Chemother* 1994;38:1490–1495.
55. Van-Poppel H, Willemen P, Wegge M, Kraseman P, Chysky V, Baert L. Antibiotic cover of transurethral maneuvers with ciprofloxacin and susceptibility behaviour of pathogens in patients with neurogenic bladder. *Urol Int* 1990;45:342–345.
56. Waites KB, Canupp KC, DeVivo MJ. Efficacy and tolerance of norfloxacin in treatment of complicated urinary tract infection in outpatients with neurogenic bladder secondary to spinal cord injury. *Urology* 1991;38:589–596.

57. Naber KG. Single-dose therapy of uncomplicated urinary infections in females: treatment of choice? *Infection* 1989;17:119–120.
58. Reid G, Bruce AW, Taylor M. Influence of three day antimicrobial therapy and lactobacillus suppositories on recurrence of urinary tract infection. *Clin Ther* 1992;14:11–16.
59. Reid G, Bruce AW, Cook RL, Llano M. Effect on the urogenital flora of antibiotic therapy for urinary tract infection. *Scand J Infect Dis* 1990;22:43–47.
60. Menge AC, Randolph JF. Fertility of spinal cord injured males: effect of genitourinary infection and bladder management on results of electroejaculation. *J Am Paraplegia Soc* 1992;15:53–59.
61. Waites KB, Canupp KC, DeVivo MJ. Eradication of urinary tract infection following spinal cord injury. *Paraplegia* 1993;31:645–652.
62. Stover SL, Lloyd LK, Waites KB, Jackson AB. Neurogenic urinary tract infection. *Neurol Clin* 1991;9:741–755.
63. Marild S, Wettergren B, Hellstrom M, Jodal U, Lincoln K, Orskov I, Orskov F, Svanborg Eden C. Bacterial virulence and inflammatory response in infants with febrile urinary tract infection or screening bacteriuria. *J Pediatr* 1988;112:348–354.
64. Menon EB, Tan EB. Pyuria: index of infection in patients with spinal cord injuries. *Br J Urol* 1992;69:144–146.
65. Peterson JR, Roth EJ. Fever, bacteriuria, pyuria in spinal cord injured patients with indwelling urethral catheters. *Arch Phys Med Rehabil* 1989;70:839–841.
66. Bakke A, Vollset SE. Risk factors for bacteriuria and clinical urinary tract infection in patients treated with clean intermittent catheterization. *J Urol* 1993;149:527–531.
67. Gribble MJ, Puterman ML. Prophylaxis of urinary tract infection in persons with recent spinal cord injury: a prospective, randomized, double-blind, placebo-controlled study of trimethoprim-sulfamethoxazole. *Am J Med* 1993;95:141–152.
68. McCue JD. Oral antibiotics: practical prescribing rules for practitioners. *Geriatrics* 1992;47:59–60, 65–66.
69. Grasela TH Jr, Paladino JA, Schentag JJ, Huepenbecker D, Rybacki J, Purcell JB, Fiedler JB. Clinical and economic impact of oral ciprofloxacin as follow-up to parenteral antibiotics. *Drug Intel Clin Phar* 1991;25:857–862.
70. Johnson HW, Anderson JD, Chambers GK, Arnold WJ, Irwin BJ, Brinton JR. A short-term study of nitrofurantoin prophylaxis in children managed with clean intermittent catheterization. *Pediatrics* 1994;93:752–755.
71. Hagberg L, Bruce AW, Reid G, Svanborg Eden C, Lincoln K, Lidin-Janson G. Colonization of the urinary tract with live bacteria from the normal fecal and urethral flora in patients with recurrent symptomatic urinary tract infections. In: Kass EH, Svanborg Eden C, eds. *Host-parasite interactions in urinary tract infections.* Chicago: University of Chicago Press; 1989:194–197.
72. Reid G, Chan RCY, Bruce AW, Costerton JW. Prevention of urinary tract infection in rats with an indigenous Lactobacillus casei strain. *Infect Immun* 1985;49:320–324.
73. Reid G, Cook RL, Hagberg L, Bruce AW. (1989) Lactobacilli as competitive colonizers of the urinary tract. In: Kass EH, Svanborg Eden C, eds. *Host-parasite interactions in urinary tract infections.* Chicago: University of Chicago Press; 1989:390–396.

Antibiotic Therapy in Urology,
edited by S. Grant Mulholland, M.D.,
Lippincott-Raven Publishers, Philadelphia © 1996.

Chapter 13

The Future of Antimicrobials

Michael Corrado

Robert Wood Johnson Pharmaceutical Institute,
Raritan, New Jersey 08869

> The treatment is simple, but requires to be put into practice vigorously...The treatment of a case of this kind must be antiphlogistic; — so far as the patient's strength will allow. The frequent application of leeches is proper; and if there be no excessive irritation, but more discharge than anything else, turpentine in small quantities has been occasionally used with advantage.... (1)

These concepts from Elliotson's *Principles and Practice of Medicine* sum up the theory and practical treatment of urogenital tract infections one century prior to the development of penicillin. One wonders how the best minds of the day could have deluded themselves into believing that leeches were proper and that turpentine could be used with advantage. In Elliotson's day, medical progress was measured over centuries, his practices differing little from those of 1744. Today, however, therapies may become outdated in a mere decade, and if not outdated, certainly less efficacious. Surveys of uropathogens from women with recurrent urinary tract infections (UTIs) demonstrate frequent resistance to trimethoprim/sulfamethoxazole (2). We have witnessed the emergence of enterococci as important nosocomial uropathogens and the potential for enterococci to acquire resistance to all known anti-infectives (3). We have observed the ability of this genetic information for pan-antimicrobial resistance to be transferred from enterococci to staphylococci and perhaps other gram-positive bacteria. And, of course, the steady acquisition of resistance to all classes of antimicrobials among gram-negative bacteria is known to all who practice the art of medicine.

It is therefore appropriate to speculate on our options. Leeches and turpentine are not among them.

In this chapter we discuss what should be, what may be, and what things we can only theorize about at present regarding new treatment modalities of urogenital tract infections.

WHAT SHOULD BE: THE NEXT 5 YEARS

There is no doubt that several of the currently useful classes of antimicrobials will have important new additions, not only in the chemical compounds themselves, but also in the way we use them.

Among the currently useful anti-infectives, over the next 5 years the greatest variety of new chemical entities will occur among the quinolones. Levofloxacin, sparfloxacin, clinifloxacin, and DU 6859a are examples of new quinolones that, by virtue of increased potency and/or superior pharmacokinetics, will be important new additions to our armamentarium. Indeed, by utilizing both of these characteristics and by dosing intelligently rather than according to historic practice, we may slow down the acquisition of resistance—the bane of our competition between humans and microbes.

Evidence both in animal (4) and, to a lesser degree, in human trials (5) suggests that anti-infectives with rapid killing potential (aminoglycosides and quinolones as opposed to β-lactams) may decrease the frequency of selection of resistance if the maximal concentration achieved exceeds the organism's minimal inhibitory concentration (MIC) by a factor of eight or more. At first blush one assumes that such is always the case, since urinary levels of quinolones usually exceed the organism's MIC by 100 times or more. But is this always true in the biofilms of foreign bodies (such as catheters), in bladder tumors with areas of focal necrosis, or in infection stones, to name a few possible sites where an organism may be exposed to concentrations less than eight times the MIC? The answer is that levels in these foci are often lacking, which probably explains why relapses and resistance acquisition occur in these and other similar settings so frequently.

By virtue of increased potency and a sufficiently broad therapeutic index, the entire daily dose of these new quinolones may be given as a single dose, thereby achieving the highest possible multiple of the organism's MIC. The long half-lives that these compounds also display ensures that urinary levels remain high throughout the dosing interval. Thus, if they prove safe in clinical trials, these new quinolones may replace most older members of the class with the theoretic potential of decreasing resistance and prolonging the utility of this entire class of compounds. Only time, measured in years, will bear out the correctness or folly of these assumptions.

Quinolones are not the only class of drugs that may be useful within the next 5 years. Research in compounds that inhibit dihydrofolate reductase (6) could lead to effective replacements for trimethoprim. Certainly new β-lactams, including cephalosporins (7), penems, and carbapenems (8), will lead to more potent, orally active compounds.

A few new classes of compounds deserve additional mention. The bioxalomycins are a new series of glycopeptides that were isolated from a streptomycete found in a soil sample from Key West, Florida. Preliminary work suggests that these compounds may inhibit DNA synthesis and that they are very active against both gram-positive and gram-negative bacteria (9).

Researchers are attempting to design compounds that inhibit the aromatic biosynthetic pathway. Since this pathway is not found in mammals, they are following the concepts of Paul Erhlich, which state that we should learn to target pathogens selectively with compounds that spare the host (10). One such hit is 6-fluro-shikimic acid. This compound, ZM 240401, is active against both gram-positive and gram-negative bacteria and was effective in protecting immunocompromised mice from bacterial challenge (11).

As a class, the tetracyclines are usually considered to be drugs whose utility in serious or "hospital"-resistant pathogens has come and gone. It is noteworthy then that a renaissance of sorts may be under way and ushered in by the glycylcyclines, derivative compounds of the older tetracyclines. These compounds have broad-based activity in vitro (12) and have demonstrated efficacy in animal models against tetracycline-resistant bacteria (13).

While traditionally one desires gram-negative coverage in a compound if it is to be useful in the treatment of urinary tract infections, the re-emergence of gram-positive bacteria as important nosocomial urinary tract pathogens requires new therapies designed to meet this challenge. The fact that many of these pathogens are resistant to current compounds suggests that if we are to be successful, we may need to look at completely novel classes of drugs. The everninomicins are an example of such a class. The everninomicins are oligosaccharide anti-infectives that appear to express bacteriostatic activity against a broad array of gram-positive bacteria. This class appears to be active against vancomycin-resistant (14) and methicillin-resistant (15) organisms.

The anti-infectives noted above are used to illustrate areas of research and to suggest some avenues researchers are exploring in order to meet challenges to our approach to the patient with urogenital infections. This is not an exhaustive overview of the panoply of chemical compounds under development, and it is by no means a litany of all that the future may hold. It does, however, demonstrate that in addition to new members of older and trusted classes of compounds, completely new classes of drugs will be important in order to keep ahead of our bacterial foes.

WHAT MAY BE: THE NEXT 10 YEARS

In 1798, Edward Jenner wrote about his observations on the cowpox (16). He noted that milkmaids infected with cowpox were immune to smallpox. Since then, medicine has ushered in a host of vaccines to a wide variety of viral and bacterial pathogens. It is not surprising that an immunologic approach to the prevention and even the treatment of urinary tract infections has long been discussed.

Vaccines with potential utility against urinary tract infections can take several paths. Monovalent vaccines are those directed against a single organism type. Such vaccines are most often used to attack a particularly problematic organism that is a common pathogen, is highly resistant to anti-infective drugs, can produce infection at a number of body sites, or that carries a high morbidity or mortality. Meitert et al. (17) described the use of a monovalent vaccine against *Pseudomonas aeruginosa*. This vaccine proved effective in protecting animals subsequently challenged with *P. aeruginosa* in up to 75% of cases for urinary tract infections. Variable protection was also obtained in respiratory, burn wound, and septicemic infection models.

Infections that do not produce significant mortality and involve a variety of antigenically distinct organisms are not economically amenable to the large series of monovalent immunizations that would be required to reduce the incidence of urinary tract infections. Infection with such organisms would be best prevented with a polyvalent vaccine.

Solcourovac is a polyvalent vaccine containing inactivated whole bacteria (18). After intramuscular injection, antibodies are produced to *Escherichia coli*, *Proteus mirabilis*, *Morganella morganii*, *Klebsiella pneumoniae*, and *Streptococcus faecalis*. Mice and rats were protected from challenge by representative strains of those bacteria contained in the vaccine. The concentration of bacteria needed on challenge to kill 50% of recipient rodents (LD50) was increased approximately fourfold for *E. coli*, *Proteus*, and *S. faecalis* and increased 600-fold for *Klebsiella*. Protection against pyelonephritis was also documented.

In another murine trial, immunization with this polvalent vaccine increased urinary IgE levels 10-fold and IgA levels twofold (19).

Human trials of Solcourovac have also demonstrated efficacy. Grischke and Ruttgers (20) studied 400 patients in an open-labeled fashion. In the 1-year follow-up period, 23 patients receiving Solcourovac developed 28 infections, while in the control group, 84 infections occurred in 47 patients.

This vaccine has been used to treat infections as well. Donovski (21) treated 25 patients with multiply resistant organisms with this preparation. Six weeks after immunization, urinary sterility was demonstrated in 68% of patients. Both of the above trials, however, suffered from lack of blinding. Large-scaled, double-blinded trials will be necessary to prove efficacy in the United States.

Since local immune responses may play an even more crucial role in urogenital tract infections, Uehling et al. (22,23) demonstrated that a multivalent vaccine administered vaginally was effective in increasing splenic antibody-forming cells directed against the organisms constituting the vaccine. Such a method of administration decreased the viability count of *E. coli* to which the animals were challenged.

While the aforementioned vaccines used a whole bacterium as the antigen, another approach is to produce immunity against an essential component of the pathogen. Since pili play an important role in colonization and invasion, vaccines have been directed against these structures.

Two types of pili, mannose-susceptible and mannose-resistant, have been shown to play different roles in the urogenital tract. Mannose-susceptible structures are those pili whose ability to adhere to the bladder can be abrogated by mannose. Indeed, it has been suggested that mannose could be utilized to block the development of cystitis (24). Once an organism gains access to the kidney proper, however, mannose-susceptible pili are repressed and a second, mannose-resistant form is expressed (25,26). In an experimental trial, Bahrani et al. (27) produced a mutant strain of *P. mirabilis* that lacked mannose-resistant pili. While the wild strain (with the ability to express such pili intact) produced higher colony counts than the mutant in the urine and bladder, the difference between wild strain and mutant was most pronounced in the kidney itself.

It is not surprising, then, that antibodies directed against pili could prove to be effective in preventing or treating urinary tract infections. Dima et al. (28) were able to protect guinea pigs successfully when challenged with a strain of *E. coli* by using a type I pilus vaccine. Dima points out that such a vaccine could have significant benefit in preventing urinary tract infections in a pediatric population. It is easy to believe that such would be the case in adults with recurrent urinary tract infections as well.

It remains to be seen whether any of these immunologic approaches will prove to be effective in larger double-blinded trials in the United States. Furthermore, it is not certain that women will avail themselves the potential protection afforded by these products. The history of adult immunizations, whether against influenza or pneumococcal pneumonia—both potentially fatal diseases—demonstrates less-than-robust participation. Indeed, often influenza immunizations must be dispensed free in order to assure some degree of participation by the public at risk. It would seem that the American archetype is historically more concerned with interventional therapy than prophylaxis.

THINGS WE CAN ONLY THEORIZE ABOUT: THE YEAR 2010 AND BEYOND

In the future we may be able to alter pathogens in most specific ways. We may be able to modify them genetically, eliminating their potential to function as parasites, replicate, or even survive by shutting down, deleting, or intentionally misinterpreting their genetic codes.

One such tool, ribozymes, are small segments of RNA that produce breaks in the normal nucleic acid sequence of a bacterium's (or virus's) RNA (29). Such breaks occur at specific sites in the organism's nucleic acid sequence. Thus, it is easy to understand that a ribozyme directed against an organism's coding sequence for pili formation, antibiotic resistance, or some essential metabolic pathway could be designed. In a simplistic sense, then, a ribozyme acts as a set of microscopic scissors that shear off parts of an organism's genetic code.

Oligonucleotides could also be inserted within or at the terminus of RNA or even DNA strands, causing a misreading of the frames and thereby leading to formation of abnormal proteins and even cell death. What will be necessary is an efficient way to introduce such forms of antisense therapy within the bacterial pathogens on a routine basis and in high-enough concentration (30). Perhaps viruses whose hosts are bacteria (phage) could be used to this end.

Such therapies directed against the integrity of the bacterium's genome are not within the foreseeable future, but work that could lead to such modalities is taking place.

If such genetic therapies are delivered using phage, it would be a precious irony, indeed, to cure human infections by promoting an infection of the bacteria themselves.

Certainly new antibacterials with advantages over those currently available will be developed. They will improve the spectrum of therapy, perhaps decrease the potential for resistance, and may be more convenient to administer. The possibilities for future vaccines are clearly workable and likely to be effective. Whether they will ever gain broad acceptance is less clear. The potential for direct genetic manipulation of uropathogens is less certain. What is clear, however, is that progressive new developments in the treatment of urologic infections are definite, will evolve rapidly over 5-year intervals, and will in each instance have advantages over all antecedent modalities.

Unlike Elliotson, we need not wait impatiently for centuries to effect changes in care and need not resort to self-deceptive practices like bloodletting in order to feel that we are offering our patients some benefit.

REFERENCES

1. Elliotson J. *The principles and practice of medicine.* 2nd ed. Philadelphia: xxxx; 1844:1004.
2. Corrado ML, Hesney M, Struble WE, et. al. Norfloxacin versus trimethoprim-sulfamethoxazole in the treatment of urinary tract Infections. *Eur Urol* 1990;34:(Suppl):17.
3. Jones RN, Erwin ME. Emerging multiply resistant enterococci (MRE) among clinical isolates: prevalence data from 97 medical centers. New Orleans: Interscience Conference on Antimicrobial Agents and Chemotherapy, 1993:abstract 1052.

4. Drusano GL, Johnson DE, Rosen M, Standiford HC. Pharmacodynamics of a fluoroquinolone antimicrobial agent in a neutropenic rat model of Pseudomonas sepsis. *Antimicrob Agents Chemother* 1993;483:37.
5. Nicolau DP, Belliveau PP, Freedman CD, Nightingale CH, Quintiliani R. Once-daily aminoglycosides: experience with 500 patients in a hospital wide program. New Orleans: Interscience Conference on Antimicrobial Agents and Chemotherapy, 1993:abstract 85.
6. Then RL, Angehrn P, Cullmann W, Hartman, P. Properties of epiroprim (RO 11-8958) as an antibacterial agent. New Orleans: Interscience Conference on Antimicrobial Agents and Chemotherapy, 1993:abstract 383.
7. Asada K, Suzuki E, Komdo N, Kuwahara-Arai K, Hiramatsu K. In vitro antimicrobial activity of a newly synthesized oral cephem antibiotic, E1100. New Orleans: Interscience Conference on Antimicrobial Agents and Chemotherapy, 1993:abstract 893.
8. Okonogi K, Iwahi T, Nakao M, Noji Y. Antibacterial activities of a new oral penem, TMA 230, and its active form, AMA-3176. New Orleans: Interscience Conference on Antimicrobial Agents and Chemotherapy, 1993:abstract 927.
9. Steinberg DA, Singh MP, Jacobus NV, Petersen PJ, Maiese WM, Greenstein M. Bioxalomycins, novel antibiotics produced by Streptomyces AP. LL-31F508: II. Biologic activities. New Orleans: Interscience Conference on Antimicrobial Agents and Chemotherapy, 1993:abstract 571.
10. Ehrlich P. Modern chemotherapy 1908. In: Brock TD, ed. *Milestones in microbiology.* Washington: American Society for Microbiology; 1975:176.
11. Davies GM, Edwards JR, Barrett-Bee KJ, Nichols WW, Wilson RG. Zeneca ZM 240401 [(6S)-6-fluro-shikimic acid]: an antibacterial agent acting on the aromatic biosynthetic pathway. New Orleans: Interscience Conference on Antimicrobial Agents and Chemotherapy, 1993:abstract 472.
12. Petersen PJ, Weiss WJ, Jacobus NV, Testa RT, Tally FP. In vitro activity of two novel glycylcycline compounds, DMG-MINO and DMG-DMDOT. New Orleans: Interscience Conference on Antimicrobial Agents and Chemotherapy, 1993:abstract 433.
13. Petersen PJ, Weiss WJ, Jacobus NV, Testa RT, Tally FP. In vivo efficacy of the glycylcyclines (DMG-MINO and DMG-DMDOT) against experimental murine infections. New Orleans: Interscience Conference on Antimicrobial Agents and Chemotherapy, 1993:abstract 442.
14. Shlaes DM, Shlaes JH, Etter L, Hare RS, Muller GH. SCH 27899 (EVE), an everninomicin active against multiply resistant enterococci and staphylococci. New Orleans: Interscience Conference on Antimicrobial Agents and Chemotherapy, 1993:abstract 460.
15. Nahashio S, Iwasawa H, Hori S, Shimada J. Comparative antimicrobial activity of everninomicin (SCH 27899), a new oligosaccharide antibiotic, against recent clinical isolates. New Orleans: Interscience Conference on Antimicrobial Agents and Chemotherapy, 1993:abstract 461.
16. Jenner E. An inquiry into the causes and effects of the variolae vacciniae, a disease discovered in some of the western counties of England, particularly Gloucestershire, and known by the name of the cow pox. 1798. In: Brock TD, ed. *Milestones in microbiology.* Washington: American Society for Microbiology; 1975:121.
17. Meitert E, Sima F, Savulian C, Petrovici M, Chersulick E, Costache G. Investigations on the efficacy of monovalent Pseudomonas aeruginosa vaccine for oral administration in Pseudomonas aeruginosa experimental infection. *Arch Roum Pathol Exp Microbiol* 1989;237:48.
18. Kruze D, Biro K, Holzbecher K, Andriai M, Bossart W. Protection by a polyvalent vaccine against challenge infection and pyelonephritis. *Urol Res* 1992;177:20.
19. Kruze D, Holzbecher K, Andriai M, Bossart W. Urinary antibody response after immunization with a vaccine against urinary tract infection. *Urol Res* 1989;361:17.
20. Grischke EM, Ruttgers H. Treatment of bacterial infections of the female urinary tract by immunization of the patients. *Urol Int* 1987;338:42.
21. Donovski L. Immunotherapy with Solco Urovac vaccine in chronic genito-urinary infection. *Khirurgiia* 1989;28:42.
22. Uehling DT, James LJ, Hopkins WJ, Balish E. Immunization against urinary tract infection with a multi-valent vaginal vaccine. *J Urol* 1991;223:146.
23. Uehling DT, Hopkins WJ, James LJ, Balish E. Vaginal immunization of monkeys against urinary tract infection with a multi-strain vaccine. *J Urol* 1994:214:151.

24. Orskov I, Ferencz A, Orskov F. Tamm-Horsfall protein or uromucoid is the normal urinary slime that traps type I fimbriated E. coli.*Lancet* 1980;887:1.
25. Kallenuis C, Molby R, Svensson SB. Occurrence of P-fimbriated E. coli in urinary tract infection. *Lancet* 1981;1369:2.
26. Leffler H, Svanborg-Eden C. Glycolipid receptors for uropathogenic E. coli binding to human erythrocytes and uroepithelial cells.*Infect Immun* 1981;920:34.
27. Bahrani FK, Massad G, Lockatell CV, et al. Construction of an MR-P fimbrial mutant of Proteus mirabilis: role in virulence in a mouse model of ascending urinary tract infection. *Infect Immun* 1994;3363:62.
28. Dima VF, Petrovici A, Dima SV, Petrovici M, Burghelea B. Immunoprotection of guinea pigs against experimental acute pyelonephritis after the administration of Escherichia coli purified fimbriae. *Arch Roum Pathol Exp Microbiol* 1989;215:48.
29. Helene C, Toulme JJ. Specific regulation of gene expression by antisense, sense and antigene nucleu acids. *Biochim Biophys Acta* 1990;99:1049.
30. Worcester Foundation for Experimental Biology. Antisense: ideal for drug resistance? *Biotech News* 1992;5:12.

Subject Index

Subject Index

ISBN 0-397-51586-3
9 780397 515868